what
to do
till the
VETERINARIAN
comes

what to do till the VETERINARIAN comes

Dr. JEAN POMMERY

with the assistance of
OTHILIE BAILLY

translated by
GLENN WEISFELD

CHILTON BOOK COMPANY
Radnor, Pennsylvania

First American Edition 1976

Copyright © 1973 by Opera Mundi.
English translation and final chapter
Copyright © 1976 by Chilton Book Company.

First Edition   *All Rights Reserved*

Published in Radnor, Pa., by Chilton Book Company
and simultaneously in Don Mills, Ont., Canada
by Thomas Nelson & Sons, Ltd.

Designed by Anne Churchman

Manufactured in the United States of America

Library of Congress Cataloging in Publication Data

Pommery, Jean.
  What to do till the veterinarian comes.

  Translation of Que faire en attendant le vétérinaire.
   1. Pets—Diseases.   2. Veterinary medicine.
I. Title.   [DNLM: 1. Veterinary medicine—Popular
works.   SF755 P787q]
SF981.P5813   636.089   75–32538
ISBN 0–8019–6298–6

234567890   432109876

►CONTENTS

v

viii   *Contents*

x   *Contents*

what
to do
till the
VETERINARIAN
comes

► DOGS

HOW SHOULD YOU SELECT YOUR DOG?

A certain charming woman of forty years had never had a dog, a cat, or even a canary. She glanced at them without seeing them. They held no interest for her—until one day when destiny arranged for her to take a trip and meet a large dog—so refined, so delicate, so well brought up, so purebred to the ends of its pedicured nails, that she was deeply touched. When it came time for her to leave him, she realized that she could no longer live without a dog. She entered the first pet shop that she saw and purchased a "darling little creature" at an exorbitant price; it died three days later. She then bought another dog that lived but which proved to be blind!

It's unfortunately true that when a person doesn't know how to select a dog or a cat, the chances are 50:50 that such a fate will befall him.

If you want to buy a dog or cat, therefore, don't run like crazy to any old pet shop because you feel you have to have a pet "immediately." That's something that no one who has raised animals for any length of time would do. Only people who have never owned pets, such as the woman above, act hastily: she had waited forty years, she could have waited another month. Besides, it's a sign of ignorance of animals to choose just any one. Even if an animal is handsome and healthy, there is no guarantee that he is right for you. It's necessary to see a lot of the animal and to wait to "fall in love" with each other before becoming "engaged."

1

There is also the matter of the Christmas present. You have promised a child, "If you are good, if you work hard . . . I'll get you a puppy." Naturally you forget about your promise. You remember on the 24th of December and race to the nearest store to buy the first pet you see. The invariable result: a horrible disappointment for the child when the animal turns out to be sick or malformed . . . or dies.

Well then, if you do want to buy a puppy or a kitten, how can you be sure that it is healthy and appealing?

It's very simple.

The puppy

If you want a purebred dog, it's in your interest to buy him from a specialized breeder. For most breeds, special kennels exist; consult your vet.

And although some pet dealers are disreputable, honest dealers can be found from whom you can get a dog in good shape.

In any case:

(1) You should examine the little creature yourself. He should be cheerful and lively, with a cold nose and a shiny coat.

If his nose is runny, he may have just a cold. But you can eliminate the risk of a viral ailment if you wait several days before buying him. If he has crusty deposits around his nostrils, beware: he is sick.

If an eye is teary, it is simply because his teeth are coming in: no danger.

If his belly is swollen and stretched like a drum, he has worms: it will be necessary to deworm him as soon as you have bought him.

If he is prostrate, lying hunched together in a corner unresponsively, he is a sick little animal.

You should not take a puppy:

(a) Whose cage is soiled by diarrhea;
(b) If there is any dried discharge at the edge of the nose, if the eyes run, or if the nose is dry;
(c) If when you pet him under the throat he begins to cough (he has a throat infection).

Lastly, have him examined by a vet within 48 hours after the purchase.

(2) A puppy must be vaccinated against certain diseases. Therefore ask to see the vaccination certificate when buying.

(3) When buying a purebred dog, inquire about his pedigree or "papers."

Now, let me give you some advice based on my experience. If you have to choose a puppy from an entire litter, I believe there is sometimes a natural affinity between a person and a particular dog. Choose without hesitation that puppy who, tripping a little over his paws and rolling around on the ground, nevertheless comes straight toward you—because it is he who has chosen you! Even if another puppy seems cuter, if he remains a little distant and observes you from across the way, don't take him. You will never come to understand one another.

Feeding a dog

Before six weeks:

If someone gives you, or you buy, a puppy less than six weeks old, he is not yet weaned and therefore should be fed with a thin mash (see the table on page 6). All regular baby foods, which you can buy at a grocery, also are perfectly suitable for a baby puppy, as long as they contain absolutely no potatoes.

After several days, add a pinch of chopped up meat to this pap. At the same time, begin to thicken it with rice which has been cooked and then rinsed.

After six weeks:

Suppose that your puppy lives with his mother. You will have begun giving him this pap for a week or two before.

After six weeks of the pap, the puppy must give up nursing once and for all. To ensure this, the mother's mammary glands must be bound.

If the puppy was separated from his mother when you bought him, he is weaned.

In either case, feeding is the same.

For several days, in order to aid the transition, offer a little reconstituted milk (see *Bottle feeding*, page 28). Gradually reduce the amount to zero.

The dog food should consist of rice or noodles (rinsed thoroughly after cooking), carrots, cooked or uncooked salads, and meat, cut up while the puppy has his milk teeth. As soon as he begins to lose them, give him a big veal or beef bone in order to expedite the process. You may add fruit to this regimen, if he is willing to eat it. If he is partial to fruit, however, don't offer too much or stomach problems may develop.

When the dog reaches adulthood, at about 18 months, stabilize the amount of food at much lower levels, especially if you live in the city. A large dog such as a German shepherd living in a city should not eat more than 10.6 to 14.2 ounces (300 to 400 grams) of red meat per day. In the country, if he exerts himself greatly— for example, a hunting dog during the hunting season—this quantity should be augmented. (Remember that because carnivores such as dogs or wolves may have to go for days without eating they have evolved the compensatory capacity to eat many pounds of meat after a successful hunt; consequently, their appetites can be enormous and are not reliable indicators of daily nutritional needs—*Trans.*)

Meat should always be either raw or very lightly grilled. The dog is a carnivore, don't forget; cooked meat, even if he likes it, doesn't suit him. Cooking risks the loss of vitamins and other nutrients.

To be avoided:

Excessive amounts of giblets, sugar, cakes, candy, chocolate— to which, alas, dogs are very partial.

To be completely forbidden:

Bones of poultry, wild fowl, lamb. Potatoes, starches, anything made from flour or meal.

Of course, the above comprises the dog's traditional diet. Nowadays, prepared dog food (dehydrated, canned, granulated) is taking over. These preparations are excellent—well-balanced and perfectly suited to dogs.

One final word of caution for the dog owner: pay close attention to the suggested quantity and don't give any more to your little bow-wow on the assumption that he is still hungry or that he is particularly fond of the day's entrée. You will soon have one fat animal!

Number of meals

When a dog reaches adulthood, it is preferable to give him a single meal per day. If you have a sensitive soul and he has eyes of quiet desperation, pretend to give him a second meal by offering him something left over from the main meal.

NOTE: If you have a watchdog or retriever, the time of his meal will vary according to his "trade."

The *watchdog* will have his principal meal in the morning; after eating, he will go to sleep. A very light evening meal will not, however, interfere with his nighttime vigilance.

The *retriever,* on the other hand, will have his big meal in the evening. It matters little if he is gorged and inert at night, so long as he is alert and lively on a day when he is in the fields.

PRACTICAL MATTERS

How to care for a dog

It is not always easy to take care of an animal. If you don't know how to approach him, he will rebel, struggle, and even, if he is not well brought up, bite.

This is what you should do:

First, it is a good idea to put the dog on a table. This has two advantages:

(1) You can work at a convenient height.
(2) His position atop a table makes him uneasy and more

DOGS

SIZE	TOY		SMALL		MEDIUM		LARGE		
Age (months)	Meat (oz.)	Vegetables and Rice or Noodles (oz.)	Meat (oz.)	Vegetables and Rice or Noodles (oz.)	Meat (oz.)	Vegetables and Rice or Noodles (oz.)	Meat (oz.)	Vegetables and Rice or Noodles (oz.)	Meals
2	1.75 (50)	1.75 (50)	2.10 (60)	2.10 (60)	3.50 (100)	3.50 (100)	5.25–7.00 (150–200)	5.25 (150)	4
3	2.10 (60)	2.10 (60)	2.45 (70)	2.45 (70)	3.85 (110)	3.85 (110)	7.00–8.75 (200–250)	7.00 (200)	3
4	2.80 (80)	2.80 (80)	3.50 (100)	3.50 (100)	5.25 (150)	5.25 (150)	8.75–12.25 (250–350)	8.75 (250)	3
5	3.15 (90)	2.80 (80)	4.55 (130)	3.50 (100)	7.00 (200)	7.00 (200)	12.25–15.75 (350–450)	10.50 (300)	2
6	3.15 (90)	3.15 (90)	4.90 (140)	4.20 (120)	8.75 (250)	7.00 (200)	14.00–19.25 (400–550)	14.00 (400)	2
7	3.15 (90)	3.15 (90)	5.25 (150)	4.20 (120)	10.25 (300)	8.75 (250)	15.75–22.75 (450–650)	17.50 (500)	2
8–12	3.50 (100)	3.15 (90)	5.60 (160)	4.20 (120)	12.25 (350)	10.50 (300)	24.50–35.00 (700–1000)	17.50 (500)	2
12–18	3.50 (100)	3.15 (90)	5.60 (160)	4.20 (120)	12.25 (350)	10.50 (300)	24.50–35.00 (700–1000)	17.50 (500)	1

Daily feeding schedule. Equivalents in grams are given in parentheses. Owners of German shepherds should figure 3.50 oz. (100 g) of meat per month of age and 2.2 lb. (1 kg) from 12 to 18 months.

tractable. If he is inclined to bite, put a muzzle on him. One can easily be made from a strap or rope:

(A) Double up the rope.

(B) Encircle the muzzle with this double-thick rope.

(C) Under the muzzle, slip the two free ends through the loop at the other end of the double-thick rope.

(D) Hold one free end in each hand and pull. The dog will not open his mouth again.

(E) Draw the ends over his neck and tie them securely.

Taking a dog's temperature

(See *Temperature*, page 103.)

How to administer a drug

Never open the dog's mouth and pour a liquid into his throat: there is the risk of his inhaling the liquid and getting a foreign-body pneumonia. Do just the opposite: close his mouth (use a muzzle if you are afraid of being bitten); then insert a syringe or eye-dropper containing the drug between his lips on the side of the muzzle, and squirt in the drug a little at a time. Simultaneously, massage the throat in order to aid swallowing.

Giving an enema

Proceed as you would with a human, except that afterwards you must grasp the dog's tail firmly in both your hands and draw it between his legs and hold it there for 12 minutes, in order to prevent immediate evacuation.

Giving a suppository

After introducing the suppository in the usual fashion, as with an enema, hold the dog's tail down between his legs for several minutes; if you don't he will quickly expel the suppository.

Getting a pill swallowed

I once knew a dog who would have thrown a fit if anyone had tried to feed him a pill by force. He insisted on taking the pill from his master's hand by himself, and swallowed it without chewing.

Not all dogs are that ingenious. However, it isn't very difficult to get them to swallow a tablet. Open the dog's mouth and press the upper lip against his teeth with your hand. That will prevent his biting—he would only bite his own lip. Now, since the entrance to the esophagus is very large, all you have to do is to hold the pill with your fingers and toss it way to the back of his throat.

How to administer a drug in powdered form

Mix it into your dog's food. If he isn't hungry, mix the powder up with a little chopped meat and feed it to him by hand.

Giving an injection

(See *Injections,* page 91.)

THE CAPTURE STICK

One evening in the country I witnessed a tragicomic episode: A large black dog had been forced against the wall of a church Growling, baring his teeth, he appeared to be crazed with fright and ready to bite the first thing that approached him.

At a respectful distance, a group of locals watched in utter fascination as an impromptu rodeo was staged: playing cowboy, a young fellow tried to lasso the miserable animal.

It was comical because of course he never succeeded. In spite of himself, he looked like one of the Marx Brothers; each time that he threw his rope like a Western hero, the youth found himself tangled up in it himself, to the accompanying laughter and wisecracks of his pals. The cowboy wound up at the end of his rope, as it were.

It was tragic because the hunted animal was so distraught that he ran back and forth to avoid the lasso.

I was offended, finding this sport cruel and idiotic.

I turned out to have been wrong in my assumption; the spectacle actually stemmed from good intentions. The dog had escaped, several days before, from a farm in a neighboring village and the youths were trying to capture him to return him. But, half dead from hunger and almost reverted to a wild state, the animal refused to let anyone approach him, which was why the attempt to lasso him had been made.

The disturbing part is that there is a difference between a cow and a dog: cattle when lassoed try to flee, while a dog at once charges the person holding the rope.

I explained this to my fine cowboy—who was glad to have an excuse to interrupt a demonstration that was beginning to make him the laughingstock of the girls!

"But how are we going to capture the dog?" one of the youths asked me.

"Bring me," I replied, "an axe handle and an old belt. I'm going to make you a capture stick—which will be easy to do."

To make a capture stick, which provides the only practical way to catch a dog disposed to bite, you need two things:

Some sort of handle . . . of an axe, a spade, or a broom.

A leather strap; a belt, for example, is fine.

Then proceed as follows:

(1) Attach one of the strap ends to one end of the handle.

(2) Fasten the sliding ring of the belt to the handle, about halfway up.

(3) Thread the belt end through this ring.

(4) Hold the free end of the belt in your hand. You thus have at your command a slip knot forming a loop adjustable to the animal's size.

(5) Holding the end of the wooden handle in one hand and the end of the freely sliding belt in the other, pass the leather loop around the neck of the dog. Draw this collar tight so that he can't get free. No matter how vicious the dog is, he cannot bite you because he is separated from you by the length of the stick. All that remains is for you to lead him wherever you want.

This capture stick can be used in the same way to handle a rebellious dog. Don't forget that a dog that is ordinarily very gentle can become temporarily crazed and vicious—from meningitis, for example.

ABSCESS

Abscesses are unusual in dogs. When two dogs fight they sometimes "devour" each other; there is no other word for it. Less subtle than the cat, they are not inclined to stop their attack when their opponent gives in. This often results in large wounds, but these bleed profusely and this is what prevents infection in most cases.

Retrievers are the dogs that most often have abscesses. They often get thorns stuck in their paws; if the thorns are not removed in time, they can cause an abscess. If so, care for the dog exactly as you would a cat. (See *Abscess*, page 122.) Dogs can have dental abscesses easily.

DENTAL ABSCESS

A dental abscess causes a swelling up toward the corner of the eye. It must be cared for like all abscesses. (See page 122.)

You should also consult a vet as quickly as possible: a rotten tooth (often caused by tartar) is responsible for the abscess. The tooth will have to be extracted and, unless you have a dentist friend who is willing to ensconce dogs and cats in his dental chair, you will need a vet for the job.

FIXATION ABSCESS

When I was the veterinarian to the king of Morocco, I went to spend a weekend with friends who owned an immense estate in the wilds of that country.

I was received like a messiah:

"I couldn't wait for you to arrive," my host told me. "The Saluki is sick and, in my opinion, he is very sick."

He led me to the dog, which was a magnificent creature of eight months, with lanky muscles and the legs of a runner. Now, however, he was huddled in a dark corner. When he spied his master, he tried to get up but he couldn't reach him.

"Have you had him vaccinated?"

"No. We are one hundred kilometers from the nearest city, and he doesn't take well to cars—well, I admit it: I put it off, put it off. . . ."

"And now he has distemper!" (See *Distemper,* page 73.)

"It's terrible. But you are going to save him, aren't you?"

I had come as a friend, not as a vet; I didn't even have my medical bag and, as my host had just mentioned, the nearest city was so far away that I could not reach it before the pharmacies closed.

Quietly and respectfully, I told him the truth: "I am very much afraid that we shall find him dead tomorrow morning."

Then something remarkable happened. You would have thought that the Saluki had heard me: he opened his big golden eyes and looked at me—how shall I say?—with such fear and at the same time such confidence that he seemed to be entreating me to save him.

But what could I do? Suddenly I remembered an old and unorthodox treatment. Having no alternative, I decided to try it.

"Have you any oil of turpentine?"

There is always plenty of it out in the country. Several minutes later, I gave the dog an injection of turpentine.

An hour later, the dog was jolted by a fit of violent shivering, howling, and panting.

His mistress asked me in a quavering voice, "Is he dying?"

"No; the fact that he is having convulsions is actually a very good sign: it shows that he is reacting. If, on the contrary, he had remained prostrate, without budging, I would have said to you, 'It's hopeless; there is nothing more that can be done.'"

The dog's masters were tortured with remorse. I left them to watch over their pet, thinking that this sleepless night was a fitting punishment for their thoughtlessness: it is criminal not to have a puppy vaccinated. As for me, I went to bed knowing that I had placed a bet in the lottery of life. Now I had to wait for 48 hours to learn whether I had won or lost.

On Sunday, the Saluki was still sick. Monday, however, at the injection site there was an abscess the size of a small grapefruit. I cut into it. (See *Abscess* in cats, page 122.)

There was one other thing: the dog's eyes were more lively and, when he saw me, he slowly wagged his tail. His instincts told him that I had saved him, for he was out of danger! His body had responded perfectly to my turpentine injection, mobilizing all its means of defense—its white blood cells—against the foreign chemical, thus effectively fighting the infection at the same time.

Let's be sure we understand this: the fixation abscess should be induced only in desperate cases of an exclusively microbial infection. It is the last means of escape when there is absolutely no alternative—neither a vet nor drugs—and when the animal is lost otherwise. This, then, is precisely how to proceed. *Do not forget this;* you may be able to save your dog with it!

(1) Sterilize a hypodermic needle by rinsing it in alcohol.

(2) Put 2 cubic centimeters (no more) of oil of turpentine into the syringe. If you have some ether, add ½ cubic centimeter of it.

(3) Make the subcutaneous injection (see *Injections,* page 91) at the top of the breastbone; that is, at the base of the neck under the muzzle. *N.B.:* Do not puncture the artery by inserting the needle too deeply!

If the animal does not respond and remains prostrate, there is no more hope; he is lost.

If he responds, he is very sick but 48 hours later the fixation abscess (which itself seems frightfully ominous) appears: the animal is saved.

You treat a fixation abscess as you would an ordinary abscess. (See *Abscess,* page 122.)

NOTE: This treatment cannot be used on cats for inducing a fixation abscess because they are highly sensitive to turpentine.

ABSCESS OF THE MAMMARY GLAND

This is very rare and only occurs if puppies are too fat and especially if they are not weaned when they begin to get their teeth. This results in a superficial abscess that is treated like that of a cat.

DOGS 13

NOTE: A tumor is often mistaken for an abscess. A mammary tumor can be recognized by these characteristics: it has an uneven, dented surface; it is not freely movable; it is very swollen, red or purple, and extremely tender. (See *Tumors,* page 108.)

AUTO ACCIDENTS

Once there was an independent sort of dog that did whatever came into her head. And her head had a distinct preference for forbidden ideas!

Thus it was that one day, in order to disobey, she crossed a street just when a truck was coming. She was seen to disappear under the wheels of the heavy vehicle. Her mistress screamed and hid her face in her hands so as not to see her pet flattened like a pancake.

A happy, excited bark made her steal a glance between her fingers. Thank heavens! The elated little darling didn't even have a scratch! The dog was shortlegged; the truck was elevated on its wheels. It had passed over her without even grazing her.

All the same, this is very unusual and usually the opposite result is produced: the little dog, like the cat, is usually killed on the spot, while a large mastiff—say, 140 pounds—makes a dent in the body of the car and limps away with a broken leg! A dog struck by a vehicle, if not killed, may have:

Fracture of the femur (upper leg bone)

This is the accident that medium-size dogs have the most often, because their thighs are at the height of a car bumper. The blow breaks the femur but at the same time flings the animal aside, which saves his life. Treat this as you do all other leg fractures, whatever the cause. (See *Fractures of the Paw,* page 61.)

Rib fracture

This occurs when the dog is hit broadside. It is very painful because it causes respiratory difficulties, especially if the broken rib ends perforate the lung. But that doesn't mean that the animal is lost. The air that is inhaled merely passes into the chest cavity and a pneumothorax results. Then the lung heals and reinflates, and everything returns to normal. If you cannot find a vet, leave things to nature and simply give the dog a sedative. (See *Sedatives,* page 39.)

If the fracture is not compound (bone piercing the skin), apply turpentine to the area and bandage it so that the dog does not lick it. This also has the advantage of immobilizing the ribs and thus forcing the dog to breathe abdominally.

Blow to the chest

This is the least serious of accidents, but compression of the thorax can lead to a form of pleuritis. Even so, nothing can be done except sedate the animal. (See *Sedatives,* page 39.)

Skull wounds

If an animal receives a blow to the head, just as with people it may be insignificant or it may be very serious and perhaps fatal. If the skull is fractured, the case enters the realm of delicate surgery. The slight chance that remains of saving the dog is to rush him to a vet as fast as possible.

If it is a case of a contusion only, it must be treated (see *Wounds,* page 95) without panicking because it is bleeding. Head wounds often bleed profusely. If the wound is very serious it must also be sutured. (See *Suturing,* page 97.)

Fracture of the toes

In many places, the law requires that dogs relieve themselves at the curb. In heavy traffic, if a driver is careless or does not like animals, his car may graze a dog's uplifted paw. Result: the paw passes under the tire, and the toes are fractured. Don't think that this is unusual; it is among the most frequent cases seen by a vet.

Go to see him at once if you are in a town. If you are far from a vet, give the dog first aid. The condition is not serious but it hurts a great deal.

Therefore you must:

(1) Administer a sedative. (See *Sedatives*, page 39.)

(2) Disinfect the wound with alcohol, or with whatever else is available instead. (See *Wounds*, page 95.)

(3) To set the fracture, apply a thick bandage, which the dog should wear for 21 days. (See *Dressing of Wounds*, page 88.)

DELIVERING PUPS

One day a wolf dog was faced with a problem: she was a film star and was about to become a mother!

That dog! She was called Youka, and everyone who saw her remembered her. She acted not from training but by using her intelligence. The director showed her in pantomime, as he would any actor, what she had to do. Her eyes followed him closely; then she repeated his actions exactly. Never was there a better canine thespian!

One day, she discovered that her human partner was performing poorly. He was supposed to kick her sharply and make her tumble to the ground. Youka, having done this previously, knew that she was supposed to fall down when his foot touched her. This she did, expertly. But the comedian didn't dare to kick this strange dog. So the animal keeled over without having been touched. When she picked herself up, she glared at the man and tossed her head back, then positioned herself in front of him again and waited for him to repeat the performance. Her eyes said clearly, "You have messed up; take it again from the top."

This was the behavior of a human being, and so astonishing that although the incident occurred more than ten years earlier, neither the director nor the comedian had forgotten it.

To return to the problem of cinematic maternity: The producer offered to remake his film rather than to give up his star. He was only doing what he would have done for Brigitte Bardot or Sophia Loren: shoot the film after the confinement.

In the morning, the dog nursed her pups—she was an excellent mother—and then she left for work. Like any mother (in France), she was permitted to return at noon to feed her infants. Like any star, she was chauffeured home in a car! She returned to the studio for three hours and then went back to attend to her pups. It should be mentioned that in her absence she entrusted them to a blue Persian, her best friend, who did not leave the pups until their mother returned. He behaved as though certain he was their father.

When this highly refined dog had given birth, there occurred all the complications that attend the confinement of an animal.

Apparently the pups were born at night, as with almost all dogs. At two o'clock in the morning I was awakened by her panicky mistress. She lived in the country and there was no point in my going out there. By the time I arrived everything would have been over. I therefore effected the confinement by telephone. For the act of birth—the most important in the life of a bitch—the animal reverted to a primitive behavior pattern. She left for the far end of a field and established herself in an impenetrable thicket where, without letting anyone know it, she had hollowed out a nest several days before.

The woman found her pet and carried the first-born pup to the house—doing just the wrong thing. Its mother of course followed!

One must always let an animal lie down at whatever spot she has chosen. Instinctively she seeks the place where she feels safe: her "nest," which she herself, and not someone else, has prepared. Now it sometimes happens, and with cats also, that the place selected is already serving as the owner's bed. I have clients who have had to relinquish their bedroom for ten days for this reason. This canine behavior reflects the ancestral instinct to protect oneself against the aggression of other animals.

"Doctor," said the mistress over the phone, "the second baby is starting to come out—my but he's cute! His head is already completely out. What do I do now?"

"Nothing!"

"But the umbilical cord. . . ."

"The dog knows perfectly well how to sever it. Be sure not to touch it, or you will provoke a disaster."

I next heard a little cry of disgust.

"She is eating the placenta!"

"And she is doing the right thing."

"Here comes a third puppy!"

"She will have at least four of them."

An instant of silence was followed by the panicky voice again: "He isn't breathing! Is he dead?"

"Not at all; he was asphyxiated by his journey from his mother's belly to the outside. Pinch his umbilical cord. He'll start to cry and his breathing will start automatically."

An exclamation of delight:

"He's breathing!"

"Return him to his mother, and don't check him every two minutes to see if he is still alive. There is nothing more to fear and you'll only drive yourself crazy!"

Silence. Then the voice again:

"Doctor, Youka has just had her sixth; she looks very wiped out."

"And you?"

"You know, I have had a child myself; it is clearly less fatiguing!"

There are times when a vet must treat a person as a simple animal and care for him as such.

"Drink a shot of whiskey," I advised. "And give a teaspoonful to Youka in a bowl of milk; she has certainly earned it! If you feel like it, you can also make her some coffee, since she would like it. Coffee is a dog's friend."

"And tea a cat's! I know, Doctor. Thank you."

I dozed off after each pup was born, cursing Youka, her panicky mistress, and the job of veterinarian. I was shaken from this irritable, somnolent state at four o'clock in the morning by a cry:

"Doctor, he is white . . . what is happening?"

I groused, "What is white?"

"The seventh puppy. Oh! He has just come out completely. He is like a little snowflake."

I had just enough energy to murmur before going back to sleep:

"Pay attention. . . ."

I heard from very, very far away, "To what?"

I answered or, more probably, thought I answered, "White wolves . . . white wolves. . . ." What was it anyway that happened to white wolves?

I slept for five minutes when the phone rang. I picked it up—no one on the line. But the ringing continued. I had to face the unwelcome truth that someone was ringing my doorbell. I opened the door to a woman whose pale face seemed to me that of a ghost and who said to me:

"I didn't dare come sooner. . . ."

"Sooner?" There are some crazy females running around at night.

Youka's mistress continued, "You must come along with me, Doctor; my dog has killed two of her pups and she is acting crazy."

All this within five minutes? That seemed absurd to me. It was then that I observed that it was eight o'clock. The young woman looked at me with the eyes of a distraught animal.

"She needs you," she told me.

Let me say that no one, even a vet, could resist Youka's commands. She was the kind of dog that one meets once in a lifetime. Colette would have said that she was "The Bitch."

Fifteen minutes later, although still half asleep, I was in Madame A.'s car, trying to comprehend what had happened:

"There was a little dog, half the size of the others."

"Scrawny?"

"Yes. When she was through giving birth, she killed him."

I reasoned that this highly civilized dog was also a wild animal and that her intelligence, fortunately, had not destroyed her primitive instincts. The latter inclinations would attempt to destroy at once a pup that was not likely to survive or that was malformed. To kill abnormal young is what she-wolves do, lionesses do. . . .

"The second?"

"He had St. Vitus's dance."

This confirmed my thesis.

"And then?"

"She went crazy. She abandoned her young and fled to a corner and howled. I felt that she did not recognize me. Only my mother succeeded in pacifying her."

There could be, I thought, two reasons for that, one exclusively medical: eclampsia. The other explanation, perhaps a product of my imagination, appealed to my interest in psychology. The dog's highly developed intelligence had rebelled against her primitive instincts and had not been able to accept the death of her young. The pulp magazines call this a "struggle of conscience." Such a confrontation had thus provoked a momentary fit of insanity.

When we arrived, the dog was lying in her bed, sides heaving, eyes staring wildly. She moaned eerily. She had the ferocious and pathetic appearance of a trapped wolf. At her side crouched an old woman who caressed her and spoke soothingly to her.

"Things are not well, Doctor," she said to me desolately. "Just now she bit the little white one—look."

On the immaculate fur there were two red scars.

What I had been trying to say when I went back to sleep came back to me.

"Be careful!" I said. "She is going to kill the white one also; almost all animals destroy their albinos. It is for this reason that nothing is more fitting than the saying 'as rare as a white wolf' or 'as a white blackbird'—birds are not exempt from this natural law either."

I extended my hand toward the pup. The hand of Madame A.'s mother caught mine in time to prevent my being bitten. The dog rose halfway out of her bed and bared her fangs but did not want to close her jaws on her nursemaid.

"Since she recognizes you, take advantage of it and remove the little one from her. Then find me a strong strap; I'm going to muzzle Youka or I won't be able to take care of her. (See *Practical Matters*, page 5.)

While I prepared a calcium injection, the mistress and grand-mistress held the white pup in their hands and fawned over him maternally. The fact was, he was the handsomest of the whole litter, and an extremely rare animal besides. On the market, white wolves are worth a small fortune!

"It's going to be necessary to separate him completely from his mother and to raise him on the bottle."

"But," the young woman protested, "without maternal warmth he will die!"

"Make a bed from a thin cushion with a hot water bottle under it so he'll always keep warm. Leave the rest to nature."

She hesitated and suggested:

"What if I gave him to the Persian to raise? He would be delighted to have a little one all his own."

I have mentioned that this blue Persian had been recruited to act as father. At the moment he was mortified: the mother, his companion, had growled at him when he had approached to admire "their" children.

The cat was sleeping curled up on the bed. We slid the little white ball between his paws. He opened his orange eyes slightly and began purring politely—then more quickly and still more quickly. He was consumed with joy. With extraordinary gentleness, the Persian clutched the pup to his silken belly and began to lick him. The cat didn't even look at us. Nothing in the world existed for him except this baby which had been given to him.

"Well and good. Now his life no longer depends solely upon you. Feed him at regular hours and he will survive."

I gazed one last time upon this touching picture which would have been worthy of inclusion in an almanac for animal lovers. This big cat was no more than four times bigger than the pup that he held between his paws and washed paternally.

"At this hour of the day the stores are still closed, but I can get milk at the farm: they are doing the milking now. I'll go get some."

The end of my story is sad, but it is animallike, the way we say something is human.

Taking advantage of her mistress' departure, abandoning her young, and opening the closed doors, Youka went up to the pup, took him from between the Persian's paws, and killed him—just like a she-wolf that will not admit having given birth to a white wolf.

Then she herself was suspended for 48 hours between life and death. She had puerperal fever.

If I hadn't been a vet, I would have said that she was dying of remorse.

I shall always remember the image of this white pup stained with red.

But I am not sure I did not suffer more agony still over this great black dog gone mad. Why not grief? Do we know anything about the psychology of animals?

I saved her. We agonized greatly over whether or not to pardon her for the death of this *Blanche*. But at the same time, I think, we became more attached to her. She was an extraordinary animal, a legendary animal. A Bosch would have portrayed her as ⅔ dog and ⅓ human.

To return to the subject of the confinement of dogs, it is important to know that it takes place after *60 days of gestation* and not 48 as many people believe. Anyway, you must:

(1) Allow the animal to give birth where she wishes. Usually two or three days before, she will begin to "make her nest" in the spot she has selected. It is always a tightly enclosed place where she feels protected against intrusions. At this time, the owner should try to set a basket or box at the place selected. It is necessary to cover the cushion or blanket with an appropriate fabric that can be removed later.

You can tell that the animal is about to deliver by noting some unmistakable signs. Her behavior becomes bizarre; she is uneasy and seeks out a corner—rarely the one you have prepared for her.

Then you must take her temperature; several hours before delivery, it falls from 101.3°F (38.5°C—normal temperature of the dog) to 98.6°F (37.0°C). This is the moment when you must anticipate everything because it is the proof that the dog will give birth during the night. Finally, there is one last symptom: just before birth, the mammary glands begin to enlarge.

(2) Delivery begins with the loss of water, which will be followed shortly thereafter (from 20 minutes to an hour) by the birth of the first pup. If all is well, the pup's head presents itself first. The other pups follow at about the same time apart. Let nature take its course. Don't interfere; let everything take place by itself.

Above all, don't interfere with the animal's eating of the placenta. It is necessary for lactation (because of the hormones it contains—*Trans.*). Moreover, it contains plenty of calcium and it is an abundance of this element that will prevent eclampsia, the convulsions due to just such a lack of calcium.

Never cut the umbilical cord. The animal knows perfectly well how to do so herself, even if this is the first time she has borne young, i.e. she is primiparous.

Lastly, it is possible that the last pup will arrive several hours after the others. This is due to the mother's fatigue and is completely normal.

However, this can produce various complications, especially if the animal is having pups for the first time.

Generally, these primiparas don't know how to manage this extraordinary series of events and are frightened. These are the dogs that seek out an enclosed nesting place most assiduously (trusting only their instincts).

Here then is how you should proceed:

(1) If the mother ignores a pup, it is useless to try to alter the facts: he is dead. In such a case, content yourself with removing him discreetly.

(2) If he is motionless but the mother doesn't abandon him, it's because he is asphyxiated. In such a case you must try to stimulate the respiratory reflex: pinch the umbilical cord sharply; this will hurt him, he will cry, and that will suffice to start him breathing. This is the equivalent of patting a newborn baby on the backside.

(3) If the pup is presented normally but the delivery is impeded, you will have to help him come out.

To do this, it is best to have two people: one massages the belly of the mother while the other takes the pup's head in his hands and pulls on it very gently while moving it up and down and from right to left.

In more serious cases, the animal may have *dystocia,* a difficult or impossible delivery. This is why, if you have a purebred animal and intend to keep her pups, it is in your interest, several days before the delivery, to have an x-ray made, which will show if everything is in order.

(1) Dystocia of volume results from the fact that the dog has been impregnated by a much larger dog; the pup's head will be too big and will not be able to pass through. If this problem is not detected before delivery, it will be readily apparent at the time of confinement: the loss of fluids will not be followed by any birth. It will then be necessary to resort to Caesarian section, which only a vet can perform. But there is no need for panic: the dog can wait for three or four days without danger to her. Obvi-

ously, however, you do run the risk of losing the pups. (See *Abortion*, page 34.)

(2) Dystocia is due to the fact that the first pup is badly positioned. I have said above that dogs are always born head first. If a pup presents otherwise, as for example sideways, he cannot come out and so he impedes the passage of all his siblings.

NOTE: It happens that certain dogs eat their young, as soon as they have given birth to them. This behavior is almost totally confined to the toy breeds. In truth, since their founding, these breeds have been abnormal: their breeders are responsible for their small size, and not nature. (A normal breed of dog should weigh at least 55 lb. (25 kg); a toy poodle, for example, is far below this.) Therefore these dogs are disturbed psychologically by their young, and they sometimes kill them.

It is unreasonable to blame the dog for this. The litter can be saved in one way: remove each pup as soon as it is born and raise it on the bottle. (See *Nursing*, page 26.)

Maladies accompanying delivery

(1) *Fatigue:* Toward the end of the delivery, especially if she has had a large litter, the dog may be very tired. If so, give her some very strong coffee with a lot of sugar.

(2) *Eclampsia:* We have already discussed this: dogs that have just given birth sometimes have convulsions of eclampsia. Whatever the cause (psychological or shortage of calcium), injection of calcium is in order. Therefore if you live far from a veterinarian, especially out in the country (Don't forget that dogs almost always give birth at night, when the vet's office is closed!), take the precaution of having some ampoules of calcium with you. You administer a calcium injection intravenously. (See *Injections*, page 91.)

Here are the dosages for a:

Large dog: 20 cubic centimeters.

Medium-sized dog: 10 cc.

Small dog: 5 cc.

Repeat the injection once a day if necessary.

(3) *Puerperal fever.* (See *Temperature*, page 103.)

(4) *Inflammation of the mammary glands.* (See *Abscess of the Mammary Gland,* page 12.) In such a case you must resort to bottle feeding. (See *Bottle Feeding,* page 28.)

Lastly, if for any reason whatsoever you decide to do away with the young, you should always nonetheless leave one of them to the mother—as much for her physiological as her psychological well-being.

If the dog is primiparous, she may become agitated and even panicky. If she does, simply give her some camomile tea which, if amply sweetened, she will probably drink by herself. This drug is a mild antispasmodic which will not interfere with the uterine contractions, but it will calm an animal.

UNDESIRABLE MATING

A client, on vacation, telephoned me, horrified:

"Doctor, it's terrible: my dog is being covered by her son! We were all in the garden and suddenly . . . how can they be separated? Should I throw some water on them?

"Don't do anything like that! If you separate them, you will cause a laceration and bleeding: the penile erectile tissue locks the male into the female and you will have to wait patiently for him to withdraw by himself."

I was aware that this disheartened woman's sense of propriety was offended by this incest. Since she couldn't see me, I didn't suppress my smile: the Oedipal complex doesn't disturb any animal! (In fact, mother-son copulations are seldom observed among primates—*Trans.*)

Back to the story.

"How old is the male?

"He's only a baby!" She was outraged at such a lack of decency. "Five months!"

"Well, it will be necessary for the dog to have an abortion. The offspring would not be pretty and of course might not even survive."

"But I am 200 kilometers away from Paris. Can I do something myself—an injection, perhaps?"

"That would accomplish absolutely nothing. There is only one way, hormone injections, and only a vet can give them. Anyway, when are you returning home?"

"In ten days."

"Well that's perfect. Bring her to me when you return. In any case it won't be possible to try anything for a good week: the time required for implantation of the egg (that is, when the fertilized egg is imbedded in the lining of the uterus)."

Don't forget this: a dog must be aborted between the eighth and the tenth day. Before is too soon, after is too late.

PUSTULOUS ACNE

If your dog loses his hair and plaques appear instead (generally between the toes), and his skin becomes grey and purple pustules appear on the plaques, he has pustulous acne. This condition is due to demodectic mange or scabies; the dog harbors a very common type of bacteria, staphylococcus (which infects the bites caused by *Demodex canis,* a mite—*Trans.*).

The following treatment therefore must be administered daily:

(1) Prick the pustules (a slightly bloody kind of liquid comes out);

(2) cauterize these with tincture of iodine;

(3) rub them with cod-liver oil.

But you must also treat the demodectic scabies which is the underlying condition; if not, the animal will never heal. (See *Demodectic Mange,* page 63.)

NOTE: Under no circumstances should you bathe the dog while he has acne.

BRUISED SOLES

That maroon poodle! He had run away from home to spend time with a female companion, and returned in the wee hours. But he didn't sneak home quietly; he could be heard whimpering from far off.

When he appeared from a field of wheat stubble (the crop having been harvested), he advanced so slowly, so pitifully, that his owners, even though they had stayed up all night waiting for him, did not have the heart to scold him.

Several hours later they telephoned me to say, "He must have injured himself because every time he tries to put weight on his paws he whines and lies down again."

I couldn't help laughing.

"That will teach him, the old stud, that one cannot chase after women without paying the consequences."

They then told me, "The wheat stubble has bruised his paws to such an extent that he has eczema. His soles—they must be all inflamed!"

"It's not serious, and you won't need a vet to treat him. Wash his soles well with a mild antiseptic."

"But we haven't any!"

"Then you have made a mistake: you should always have one when you own animals. Well then, have you any copper sulfate?"

"No, but my neighbor is a wine-grower; he'll have some for sure!"

"Go and ask him for five grams which you will mix in one quart (a little less than one liter) of boiled water and clean your poodle's paws with it. Actually it's a powerful astringent which will harden the natural callosities. But be sure that your dog doesn't lick himself, or he'll be poisoned! Afterwards apply some vaseline or, if you have none, some lard to his soles and in two days he will be cured."

NURSING

Miriam lived in a dog pound. Her tribulations would have been worthy of a dime novel in the 1890's tradition of *Seduced and Abandoned*.

She was a beautiful animal, half sheepdog and half wolf, with a gentle and optimistic demeanor that all the pitfalls of life had not made her lose.

The owner of a suburban house had found her one day, starving, at her door. She herself owned a strong, handsome, "pure-bred" German shepherd, she said with pride. She shoved a bowl of leftover soup toward this wayward dog but did not permit this "bastard" to so much as enter her house. Appreciative of that much kindness, the animal lay down before the gate and, wagging her tail amiably, waited for someone to throw her the remains of the handsome male's meal. The latter played the role of a grand duke; he used his noble bearing to seduce the unfortunate waif. When she got pregnant, the indignant mistress decided to drive this good-for-nothing to the pound. To take her there, since the woman did not want to touch such a flea-ridden animal to put a collar on her, she went outside with the male. Humbly, trotting behind him, the animal followed her mate. He led her straight to the animal refuge. That proved to be her first break in life! The keeper, an honorable man affected by genuine pity, found her a good owner.

It was they who, several weeks later, called me, the dog having presented them with an unexpected gift: 12 pups!

I found the mother ensconced in an immense basket, her young hanging to her teats. It was the happy ending of romance magazines! She seemed very contented and satisfied with herself. I myself was much less pleased: the babies sucking at the teats were all trying to cry more loudly than the next.

"Just look at them!" the mistress gushed. "What a marvelous picture!"

I wasn't so enraptured.

"A picture of pups dying of hunger! Personally, I find this scene more suggestive of the *Raft of the Medusa*."

Mrs. B. looked at me in horror.

"But Doctor, they are sucking!"

"Yes, but they are sucking up nothing!"

I held the two last mammary glands.

"See, these are slack and don't contain a drop of milk!"

"Maybe those two; but there are six others."

That's true; a dog has from six to ten mammary glands. However, there is one very important thing to know: lactation is mediated almost exclusively by the two inguinal mammary glands; that is, the last two. Although identical in appearance to these two, the others are almost useless. Whenever you see puppies clinging to them, say to yourself that they are the equivalent of a baby's rubber nipple. That's why it is necessary to oversee the process of nursing, even if lactation is normal. Two puppies are always smarter than the others and get hold of the "bottles" and monopolize them. It's your responsibility to remove them when they have had their fill and to install the other nurselings alternately in their place, if you want the entire litter to be nourished adequately.

But in this case, something was more serious: as soon as I had heard the pups whine, I was certain that they were hungry: a baby, whether human or animal, only cries if he has a reason for doing so. And to eat is the most important reason.

Miriam's unhappy experiences doubtless were responsible for her lack of milk.

"What am I going to do?" my client asked me.

"Bottle-feed them, of course!"

And that's what she did—and very successfully.

Well then, don't forget, in a case of:

Normal lactation

All or almost all lactation occurs through the posterior mammary glands. Now it often occurs that during and soon after delivery the mammary glands are extremely hard. The pups naturally try to make things easy on themselves: they hurry over to the more supple teats—which contain nothing. You have to massage the inguinal mammary glands gently, draw out the first drops of milk, and then force the young to attach themselves to these teats. Once the mammary glands are decongested, you will have no problem except to see that each pup receives his full ration.

Bottle-feeding

If the mother has no milk, it will be necessary to bottle-feed the pups. If the dog has more than six young, it will also be necessary to consider, in advance, the possibility of bottle-feeding to make up the difference.

You will be able to tell that the animal has no milk by observing the pups.

Immediately after nursing, a puppy goes to sleep. If, contrary to this law of nature, he cries, is agitated, and goes from one teat to the other, check the mammary glands. If they are flaccid and if, when you pinch the ends, no milk spurts out, this indicates that your fears are well founded.

If so, proceed at once to bottle-feeding.

For this:

(1) Find a bottle; a normal baby bottle is perfect for the young of large dogs. For the pups of the toy breeds (and for kittens), a doll's baby bottle is preferable; the nipple of a regular baby bottle is too large for these pups to take in their muzzles. Starting from the first day, the food of a puppy must be nutritious. It is made up of the following mixture:

An egg, or just the yolk, beaten in one ounce (30 grams) of milk. If the puppy can consume two ounces, fold in two eggs, etc. But better still, if you have the opportunity, go to a pharmacist who sells powdered dog's milk.

NOTE: I have observed that most of my clients do just the opposite of what this regimen calls for: they give their puppies cow's milk, sweetened with sugar and diluted with water. This is tantamount to condemning the little animal to death. Dog's milk, if less sweet than cow's milk, is in fact much richer; it takes 40 days for a calf to double its weight and 8 days for a puppy to do so.

(2) Fill your bottle and give it to the pup. At first you may have a little trouble; he may not want to take this nipple which to him is not natural. You will have to force it on him; he will become accustomed to it very quickly.

Allow him to drink as much as he wants. A little animal never exceeds his capacity. Then return him to his mother so he can go to sleep against her warm body.

(3) Repeat this routine nine times per day. Obviously, even if you have only six pups to raise, your days will be plenty busy! But these nine nursings are absolutely mandatory to assure the life of the nurseling.

(4) At the end of three weeks you will be able to begin to wean the puppy. (See *Feeding a dog,* page 3.)

JUVENILE ANASARCOID

Blond, petite, haughty, the young dachshund was perfectly suited to her blond, sophisticated mistress, who was the wife of a general. Both of them acted as though the world existed only for them. And they admired each other with eyes of an identical hazel color.

Imagine her horror, then, when the general's wife arose one morning to find her glamorous pet transformed into a shapeless ball. The dog's eyes, ears, and paws had doubled in size—and "stuff" was running out. The adorable thing had changed into a little repulsive monster that she brought to me in sorrow. The two of them had lost all of their haughtiness!

"What shall we do, Doctor?" wailed the young woman. "Are you going to have to give her an injection?" she asked, genuinely in anguish over her dog.

I began to laugh.

"I believe that you have a son and that he has had acne recently. Well, your dog has juvenile anasarcoid."

The juvenile and familial aspects of the condition reassured her and, in fact, several days later the dog had become svelte, petite, and again haughty!

Juvenile anasarcoid is an illness of puppies; adult dogs never get it.

The symptoms are those that I have just described; it is a sort of hives which appears with a remarkable rapidity. We think that it is due to a staphylococcus infection and so it is treated with antibiotics.

If, one morning, you suddenly notice that your puppy has this condition and if you cannot get to the vet immediately, here is the emergency treatment to be administered in the meantime:

(1) Wash all the swollen and oozing areas with a mild disinfectant. This will also act as an astringent and begin to dry the skin.

(2) Apply a sulfurous ointment to the affected areas. If you have none, mix equal parts of hog's lard (melted pork fat) and flowers of sulfur.

(3) Every day give the animal two good tablespoons of brewer's yeast (obtainable from any pharmacist).

Even after all this, take the puppy to the vet as soon as you can, because the antibiotic therapy can only be prescribed by him and is indispensable for a complete cure.

ANGINA (OF THE THROAT)

There are two types of angina:

First, the kind a human has and transmits to his dog. In such a situation, both patients are cared for together and in the same manner: daubing of the throat, aspirin—not too much for the dog (see *Sedatives,* page 39) but external application of tincture of iodine, and—why not?—a nice mixture of lemon and honey like his master gets, which he will lap up eagerly because the honey is sweet. Then both patients should snuggle up in bed and wait for the illness to pass.

Then there is the other kind of angina. This is no trifle; it is caused by a virus. You will notice this condition when your dog has trouble swallowing; you will have the impression that he has tried to swallow something that won't go down all the way. But if he can eat, there is no foreign body that is preventing him from swallowing.

If your dog is young and has not been vaccinated, go to a vet at once: distemper always begins in this fashion. This type of angina obviously can be a consequence of the eruption of the teeth, but only a qualified person can make this differential diagnosis and if you delay going to him, you may be too late!

ARTHRITIS

Walter was a French pointer, a great retriever without parallel in flushing a partridge or dislodging a hare.

At the end of a day of hunting on which he had been worked especially hard, he returned home limping badly.

His master, searching vainly for a thorn which might have injured him, noticed that the animal whimpered when he took its paw.

He telephoned me.

"I am sure he has arthritis," I told him. "Feel the joint and see if it is warm and slightly swollen."

This was indeed the case.

The owner suggested, "I am going to apply some warm compresses; that will soothe him until I can take him to you."

"That's the worst thing you could do! The heat would increase the inflammation of the joint and your dog would just suffer all the more. To the contrary, apply very cold compresses, or better yet, soak the affected paw. Then apply a plaster of vinegar and whiting, and wrap the whole paw securely with an elastic bandage. And of course don't take him hunting tomorrow. And when you return to Paris bring him to me because this procedure should be followed by antibiotic treatment."

Arthritis is in fact due to an inflammation of a joint which has been strained or shocked. It is the invasion of some microbe (hence the antibiotic therapy) of the strained joint which leads to the arthritis. To treat it:

(1) Minimize the inflammation with cold, by applying ice water compresses to the joint or, better still, by using running water. A garden hose works perfectly.

(2) Massage the paw.

(3) Prepare a plaster out of equal parts vinegar and whiting, and apply it to the joint. This astringent will also aid the process of decongestion.

(4) Dress the whole paw (See *Dressing of Wounds,* page 88) with an elastic bandage.

Allow the animal to rest, of course, and repeat the treatment until he is no longer limping.

ASPHYXIATION

In the last century, the Duke of York was renowned for his coal mines which were themselves famous, unfortunately, for their tragic "firedamp explosions."

The miners used dogs to detect the toxic gas. Closer to the ground than man, the dog would be asphyxiated before the miner was. Thus if a miner saw a dog collapse in front of him, he knew the deadly gas was present and he had no choice but to flee as fast as his legs would carry him. However, dogs were forbidden in the mines.

So the clever miners got the smallest dogs they could find in order to be able to hide them under their jackets.

Bantering casually, they passed before the employee who checked them over at the entrance. Their hands were in their pockets—and their dogs hidden against their chests. Once down in the mine, they released the little animals whose job it was to save their lives.

Entertainment was hard to come by in an age without television or films. Getting together at a pub on Sundays, the miners compared their little friends, weighing them to determine their differences in weight, to see who had the smallest and cutest dog. The gambling and sporting spirit of the Anglo-Saxons was aroused; contests were organized. In order to win, the miners took up the practice of breeding, to obtain smaller and smaller and more and more handsome specimens.

In this way the Yorkshire breed was founded.

I have brought this up in order to emphasize that an animal can be asphyxiated more easily than a man. Escaping gas can cause the death of a cat or a dog, all the more quickly if he is small.

If an animal is asphyxiated, don't lose any time in calling a vet. It isn't he who will save your pet but the quickness of your reflexes. The other steps to take in such a case are the same as for a man:

(1) Immediately carry the dog into another room and place him before a wide open window. If he doesn't come around at once, you must:

(2) Give "mouth-to-muzzle" respiration! Obviously it is impossible to give mouth-to-mouth resuscitation to a dog or any other animal—his large snout won't retain the air! Here is how to proceed:

(a) If it bothers you to have your mouth in contact with the animal's muzzle, place a very fine handkerchief or gauze bandage—something that air can pass through—over the muzzle.

(b) Inhale and exhale in accordance with your own respiratory rate—about 16 times per minute.

(c) Massage the dog's chest to the same rhythm. This will help prompt the resumption of breathing and will also facilitate the heart's beating, or help it resume beating if it has stopped. (See *Cardiac Massage*, page 81.)

NOTE: Sometimes at the conclusion of resuscitation the dog's stomach is filled with air. If so, press on his stomach to expel the air. If you don't, just the opposite of the intended result may occur: in trying to save the animal you may suffocate him.

As a matter of fact, the enormous capacity of a dog's stomach can compress the diaphragm and increase the risk of asphyxiation.

So it is best, when you are finished, to bandage the whole thorax, from behind the front legs to the last ribs, so that air which collects in the stomach will be forced to go into the lungs.

When the dog has recovered his senses give him some strong, sweetened coffee to aid his heart (for a cat, tea without sugar).

When the dog begins to breathe again, if you happen to have a tank of oxygen, give him some to breathe for several minutes. (See *Lack of Oxygen*, page 87.)

Finally, if possible, let a vet examine him anyway.

ASTHMA

In fact, asthma does not occur in dogs. (See *Bronchitis*, page 35.) But allergies exist that resemble asthma in that breathing is impaired, especially allergies due to certain pollens, modern fabrics, and, very commonly, feathers. (See *Hives*, page 111.)

ABORTION

This is perfectly legal and is often essential—as, for example, when a female cocker spaniel falls in love with a big setter.

If pups result from such a union, the mother will have a difficult delivery. (See *Dystocia*, page 55.) This calls for a Caesarian section.

So if such a situation develops, it is much better not to wait for the births but rather to take the dog to the vet eight to ten days after copulation. (See *Undesirable Mating*, page 24.)

BALANOPOSTHILITIS

This is an inflammation of the penis and the foreskin. A dog with this condition licks his penis cautiously but persistently.

Sometimes a small amount of secretion which has the appearance of pus is visible at the end of the foreskin. A case of this kind calls for thorough rinsing with a standard gynecological solution (which you can ask the pharmacist to prepare for you). Use a small eyedropper; insert the tip under the foreskin.

BRONCHITIS

His whole family having had the flu, Merlin the fox caught it in turn. He coughed as much as did his two-legged father, mother, and brother, and he whined and was completely prostrate. Since the people were confined to their rooms, there was no way of taking Merlin to the vet, so they treated him in the same manner as themselves. They were indeed correct!

Don't forget: Bronchitis, the flu, and the common cold of man can be contracted by animals.

Therefore, take the same precautions toward the animal that you would toward a child: don't kiss him, don't take him onto your lap, don't let him near your handkerchiefs.

If, however, whether or not through a fault of your own, your pet gets bronchitis, this is how to care for him:

(1) Give him an inhalant. (See *Common Cold in Cats,* page 138.)

(2) Give him a turpentine rubdown on his chest. NOTE: This is only for dogs; be sure not to do this to a cat, which won't be able to stand it.

(3) Take his temperature. If he is feverish (See *Temperature,* page 103) give him a very tiny bit of aspirin; don't exceed the dosages that I have prescribed. (See *Sedatives,* page 39.)

(4) Give him suppositories with a eucalyptus base.

The dosages for animals are always the same regardless of the particular drug:

Large dog: adult dose.
Medium dog: child's dose.
Small dog: baby's or cat's dose.

(5) Lastly, if you have cough syrup, make him take it according to the same regimen.

NOTE: Chronic bronchitis can only be treated by a vet.

Bronchitis in a puppy

You have to be careful because often it's not really bronchitis even though the puppy is coughing.

In reality it may be:

(1) the onset of distemper or some other viral illness;
(2) due to the passage of ascaris larvae into the bronchi. (See *Worms*, page 113.)

BURNS

More and more, veterinary medicine resembles human medicine; we treat our four-legged friends with the same medications and the same procedures as ourselves.

In his book *What To Do Till the Doctor Comes*, Pierre Fournier recommends treating burns by putting the affected area under a faucet of cold water for a quarter to a half hour. Tap water is best because its temperature is cool and it is chlorinated. The idea behind this is:

to ease the pain
to chill the burned area
to inhibit swelling
to prevent painful blisters from forming.

Lastly, if the burn is slight, wrap it with sterile linen; it will heal by itself.

I wouldn't add or substitute another thing: this procedure is as useful for animals as for people.

If the burn is serious take your pet to the vet as fast as possible, just as you would take a burn victim to a hospital.

However if it is only that you don't have any running water at your disposal, as often happens in the country and when camping, follow this alternate procedure: pour alcohol at a temperature of about 175° (80°C) on the burn. This seems shocking, but it was recommended by my professor at the Veterinary School of Toulouse and my experience has convinced me of its efficacy. The alcohol disinfects and at the same time "tans" the skin. It has, however, the disadvantage of temporarily aggravating the pain of the burn.

Lastly, if you own some land or if you are camping near some oak trees, there is yet a third solution which can be substituted for the other two. Take a big piece of oak bark and boil it in water for half an hour. Allow this decoction to cool and use it to apply compresses to the burn. The tannic acid in the bark passes into the water and dries the wound.

Animals can have a complication that does not exist with humans: fur. Once burned, the fur falls out, a scab forms on the wound, and it is absolutely necessary to remove the hair in order to prevent infection. Now if you content yourself with pulling it out, not only will you be hard pressed to get it all, but the poor animal will suffer horribly. Therefore use cod-liver oil for this purpose. It's an excellent emollient which, furthermore, aids tissue repair. You pour some onto a compress which you then pass gently over the bunch of hair until you have succeeded in cleaning the burn completely.

You can also use pharmaceutical oleocalcareous liniment. It's an excellent old remedy which works as well on cats as on dogs. Take about 28 ounces (100 g) of lime water (see under *Diarrhea in a puppy*, page 74), and the same amount of olive oil.

Shake vigorously until thoroughly mixed.

Smear the burn with this liniment. Repeat three or four times a day until healing is complete.

CHEMICAL BURNS

Fire and boiling water aren't the only things that cause burns.

The little "darling" that was brought to me one day was crying as though he were flayed alive—and he almost had been. Tempted by curiosity—a dangerous character flaw—he wasn't satisfied until he had knocked over a bottle to see what it contained: smelling salts! The poor dog had his four paws frightfully burned. Such accidents happen often, especially in the country. In such a case you should:

(1) wash the wound thoroughly with water to rinse out the acid.

(2) treat the burn with a chemical opposite to the kind that caused it, that is:

Acid Burns

Hydrochloric or sulfuric acid burns are healed by alkaline substances; the simplest of these is one found in every home: soap. So if an animal burns himself with any sort of acid, lather him with soapy water.

NOTE: Use a very mild soap: household soap that you grate into little pieces, or soap flakes that you dissolve, a handful at a time, in a bowl of water.

You can also use baking soda (one tablespoon in a glass of water) or mineral water.

Alkaline burns

(Caustic soda, ammonia, and certain very strong lyes used to wash walls): treat these with acidic solutions. Here again you can use a very simple remedy: vinegar.

ELECTRICAL BURNS

He was called Sonny because he was an exact copy, hair for hair, of his mother: a black Alsatian with a muzzle the color of dead leaves.

He was five months old and he spent all his time trying to think up new brands of mischief.

One day he discovered an electric cord. It fascinated him, all the more because his master forbade him several times to touch it. His aggressive spirit became aroused and, when his master ·vas out of the room, he seized the cord between his teeth and began to chew joyously.

The cord avenged itself: it burned Sonny's tongue and lips. He yelped and went to seek protection from his master who, after all, hadn't been so wrong! After the customary "I told you so," Sonny's master set about the job of treating him. Since he didn't know exactly how to go about it, he first disinfected the wound with hydrogen peroxide and then brought the dog to me.

But the wounds were superficial and so I couldn't improve on what he had done.

So, in a case of a slight electrical burn, disinfect it with hydrogen peroxide and leave the rest to nature.

SEDATIVES

All the sedatives used for humans, including barbiturates, are effective for dogs.

The only one to distrust is . . . aspirin!

There are two reasons:

(1) Aspirin harms the kidneys. In man—unless he abuses the drug—this is of little significance. In the dog, however, the kidney is a most important and fragile organ, and therefore aspirin can cause very serious problems. For this reason, if you have nothing else to give, under no circumstances exceed a dose of one to two tablets for a large dog, and one tablet for a small dog. But above all, don't continue it for more than three days. If the aspirin is still needed, wait for 48 hours before resuming it.

(2) In case of a wound: aspirin is also an anticoagulant, so it can aggravate bleeding.

With regard to the other analgesics, here are the dosages to abide by for an adult animal.

Large dog: about 65 pounds (30 kg) or more, such as German shepherd, greyhound, Great Dane, mastiff—the same dose as for a man.

Medium-sized dog: about 20 to 55 pounds (10 to 25 kg), such as French pointer, spaniel, medium-sized schnauzer, etc.—the same dose as for a child.

Small dog: about 2 to 20 pounds (1 to 10 kg), such as toy poodle, Yorkshire, dachshund, etc.—the same dose as for a baby.

MAD DOG

This isn't an illness, you may say. But it may be one: rabies. It can also be a symptom of a physiological—or psychological—malady. Dogs, like people, have their mental states!

Here are these three possibilities in a single case history.

Some time ago a gypsy brought me a very handsome dachshund of about 12 months of age. The dog was a "biter." He had attacked an inoffensive passer-by and therefore had to submit to the established prophylactic procedures for rabies. (See *Rabies,* page 99.) For the dachshund this consisted of visits to the vet every day for three weeks.

I must say that when he entered my office, I had never seen a more aggressive dog. The first thing I did was to muzzle him. Then I set him on the examining table and palpated him. I felt something hard in the digestive tract.

"I don't know if he has rabies, but he definitely has an intestinal obstruction and his suffering is probably the cause of his bad temper. How long has it been since he had a bowel movement?"

"Oh," replied the gypsy, "eight, ten days. . . ."

"Then this calls for emergency surgery."

It is important of course to try to prevent, to the extent that it is possible, the death of a dog that is suspected of having rabies.

I opened the stomach of the dog and what should I find but a peach stone! (See *Peach stones,* page 48.)

I removed the pit and closed up the incision. Everything was going fine except that, in the evening, my gypsy forgot to return to retrieve his dog! So I left the dog in my office overnight. Then when I returned the next morning to enter my office—it was impossible. The dachshund had been transformed into a ferocious little monster and refused to let me in. I was forced to employ a capture stick. (See *The Capture Stick,* page 8.) Then I locked him in the kennel where I kept animals after surgery, while I awaited his master. The day passed, and again no gypsy.

In the evening when I brought this mad dog his dinner before I left, he curled his lips and his eyes were filled with terror at the mere presence of a human being.

The next day, and the day after that, still no gypsy. It was time to acknowledge the obvious: he had found it convenient to abandon a dog that had caused him so much trouble.

The dachshund himself no longer growled. On the third day he even went so far as to wag his tail when I opened the door of my office. So I let him run loose. On the eighth day when I removed his stitches, not only did he not protest but he gave me such a trusting look that I was bowled over by it.

What should I have done? I kept him from escaping, to be sure. But he was the gentlest, most affectionate dog that I had ever had. His physical suffering alone and, from all appearances, his fear of his first master, had made him into a mad dog. It is hardly necessary to say that he didn't have rabies.

So if you own or know of a bad-tempered dog, always remember that rabies is very unlikely—his ill humor probably indicates an ailment or simply unhappiness.

COLIC

See *Worms,* page 113.

CONSTIPATION

It was a Sunday. The dog hadn't had a bowel movement for a whole week and his owners had taken him into the country, thinking that the grass and the freedom would help him defecate.

They thought that they had hit on the right strategy. Medor galloped off and ran three laps around the field, and then he got into position. But this produced nothing but a long wail of pain. He tried again, with the same result. Then, resigned, he gave up, after having glared angrily for a long time at his recalcitrant anus.

His master, concerned, examined it also. He noticed a kind of hard ball that was obstructing the opening. Then he recalled that Medor had eaten a lot of bones that week. He concluded, logically enough, that these pieces of bone had formed a barrier at the level of the rectum, preventing defecation totally.

What was to be done?

The owner remembered that when he had been a child, his grandmother used to cut out a little triangle from a bar of soap and give it to him as a suppository. The results were always rapid and perfect.

He decided to do the same thing for Medor, which was an excellent idea. Unfortunately, the bunch of bones blocked the anus in both directions and he was not able to introduce the suppository.

Then, taking a small stick, he set about the task of breaking apart this bony plug. With much patience he finally succeeded and, thus disencumbered, Medoc was able to conduct his business.

There is no other solution, no matter how disagreeable it may seem to you.

When a dog's constipation is due to an obstruction of bones:

(1) Make a suppository out of soap and introduce it into the rectum. If you succeed in doing so, this will probably be sufficient.

(2) If not, after lubricating the anus with oil, put on a rubber glove and insert your finger (or use a little piece of wood) into the dog's rectum and break up the mass of bony debris.

Don't let this condition go uncorrected, or it will lead inexorably to intestinal occlusion and a serious operation.

If a dog is habitually constipated (and that happens easily, because dogs have delicate livers), administer a tablespoon of linseed, castor or paraffin oil (see *Feeding a dog*, page 3). NOTE: Never give him a laxative for humans, especially one with a calomel base.

Avoid like the plague the old wives' remedy of making the dog swallow a handful of salt, under the generally mistaken assumption that he is poisoned. For some mysterious reason, salt has been regarded as a universal panacea by peasants for several centuries. It is, in fact, extremely dangerous for animals.

Thus I was once summoned to a farm in an "extreme emergency," which certainly was the case, since the dog had died by the time I could get there.

"Alas," the fellow sighed, saddened by the death of his pet, "I did what I was supposed to, Doctor. Since he wasn't moving his bowels, I thought that he had been poisoned, so I gave him a big spoonful of salt. And when that didn't work I made him take some of my own medicine."

And he proudly showed me a box of calomel.

Now salt, combined with calomel, produces a mercury salt that is fatal.

In trying to cure him, my well-intentioned peasant had killed his dog!

FOREIGN BODIES

In the throat

I have already told you about Youka, that extraordinary German shepherd. One day while her owners were finishing lunch, they saw her enter the kitchen.

"Her behavior," they told me later, "was so strange that we understood at once that something serious had happened. She sat down before us and looked at us with such intensity that somehow she caught our attention. She foamed a little at the lips, and she panted; but she wasn't panicky. Immobile, she remained before us, waiting—that was apparent—for Man to come to her rescue.

The maid confessed in a quavering voice, "I gave her a goose bone and I think it has caught in her throat." This clarified the situation but did not make it any less dramatic.

While the master telephoned me (But what could I do? By the time I arrived, the animal would be dead!), the mistress had opened Youka's mouth and, feeling around with her fingers, tried to locate the piece of bone that was stuck in the dog's throat.

"It was incredible," she related. "I didn't even have to hold her mouth; she kept it open by herself. She didn't budge but paid close attention to my slightest movement. You might have said that she was engrossed in the effort to save her life, just as I was.

But she was choking, and a white foam was accumulating around her lips. And her eyes, which had become slightly glassy, never left me. They seemed to say, 'Hurry, I am suffocating, I shall die if you don't remove that bone which is killing me.' And then, suddenly, her eyes expressed insufferable emotion! It was the end. Desperately I plunged my hand in still deeper and I felt something hard; I pulled gently on the end of the broken bone the way you would on a bevel that had been wedged in between two pieces of wood. . . ."

If something like this happens to you, don't waste any time. Do exactly what Youka's mistress did. It is the only way to save your dog.

When a foreign object gets lodged in the larynx and blocks the passage of air, edema occurs instantaneously. This envelops the bone or whatever, causing total blockage of the passage of air. Unable to breathe, the animal dies in several minutes.

Don't forget: to save your pet's life, stick your hand right into the dog's throat and pull out the bone that is lodged there. Don't waste a second or wait for a vet, who will only arrive too late!

In the mouth

The little schnauzer seemed to have gone crazy. He whimpered all the time, or he stopped abruptly and began to rub his muzzle with his two front paws as if he were trying to wear it away, or else he shook his head as though he had decided to get rid of it.

"My God, what has happened to him?" wailed his mistress. "At least he doesn't have rabies, does he, Doctor?"

I explained to her that this behavior, although strange, had nothing to do with rabies but could very well be due to a fragment of ordinary wood.

I opened the animal's mouth. As a matter of fact, a little branch had gotten wedged in the upper jaw and covered the whole palate, and the dog was trying unsuccessfully to dislodge it—hence the bizarre St. Vitus' dance.

If you ever observe your own dog so affected, before doing anything else open his mouth and see if a piece of wood or bone is stuck in his jaw.

I often instruct a client to open the animal's jaws, but am frequently told, "Oh, I don't dare; I'm afraid he'll bite me!"

In such cases it isn't the dog which deserves punishment, but the master!

A dog should never bite anyone *especially not his master*. If he does so, it's because he has been poorly trained. Every puppy should be taught that its master has the right to place his hand between its teeth, and it does not have the right to close its teeth on that hand. There is a very simple way to make a dog understand this. When he is still a puppy, give him a beef bone, wait until he has begun to chew on it, and then advance your hand to take it from him. If he growls at you, give him a light tap on the muzzle and draw the bone away from him. Then return it to him and pet him reassuringly; then repeat the procedure until he understands.

This is very important! If Youka hadn't learned to allow this kind of handling, she would have been dead.

"Potatoes" in the ears

This could be the title of a surrealistic novel. Actually, these "potatoes" are a particular wild grain that children sometimes slip into their sleeves in order to enjoy having them run down their arms.

During the hunting season dogs, especially those with long ears, pick these things up—unintentionally! The "potatoes" enter the ear of the unfortunate setter or spaniel and "run down" the auditory canal as easily as they do a child's sleeve.

The dog goes crazy and his master is usually convinced that he has meningitis! Actually, this invasion of his ear makes the dog lose his sense of equilibrium, and he walks around with his head tilted until he falls down or rolls around on the ground trying to rid himself of his "potato." This calls for removal of the grain at once, which isn't easy. If you can see it, trap it with a pair of tweezers and remove it. But don't try to do this with your finger —you'll just wedge it in farther. If it has disappeared completely, it becomes exceedingly difficult to locate. Furthermore there is the risk of otitis. (See *Ear Ailments*, page 83.)

Broken glass and needles

Little dogs are like little children: they only know how to think up mischievous pranks. If they are intelligent they will, very cleverly, do their mischief-making on the sly.

Thus I once knew a young Airedale who posed a real enigma to one of my clients.

The owner kept on his bureau one of these stuffed animals that were popular some years ago: a little furry seal with two black-headed pins for eyes. The Airdale adored this seal and one day when Mr. D. had gone out, the dog took the seal gently in its lips and played with this doll, without damaging it. When the master returned he found the little seal, wet with saliva, on the floor, just as he might have found some baby's toy. And next to the seal were the two black-headed pins which the dog had very delicately removed from the seal's head. Why? That was a question that the owner hoped he would never have to answer.

This detail troubled Mr. D., who was afraid, quite reasonably, that the animal might very easily swallow one of the pins while playing. Therefore he warned the Airdale sternly to exercise self-restraint over the matter of the seal.

Several days later, the master returned home and found the little plaything perched on the mantelpiece. Mechanically he reached for it to put it back in its place. Then he noticed that its eyes were missing. He looked on the floor: they were there. Despite the Airedale's intelligence, it was hard to believe that he had been able to carry the seal to the mantelpiece. The master decided to conduct an experiment: seal and dog were left alone in the room. And the master was compelled to yield to the empirical conclusion: every time he tried this, he found the little toy on the mantelpiece with its eyes missing.

The Airedale, knowing that this was wrong for him to do, always replaced his toy so as not to be punished. Sometimes he got the mantelpiece and the bureau mixed up, but he didn't think that this was serious and he was certain that his master wouldn't notice—but he forgot about the eyes that he had removed!

Another dog, a young German shepherd living in a village, once organized a burglary.

One day the dog's caretaker had to spend the afternoon in town. She told the pet to mind his manners and then left.

In the evening she returned and, opening the door, beheld a shocking scene. On the table was a crudely set place, with everything necessary for a meal: a glass, a piece of bread, an open jar of preserves. She immediately thought of a burglary, since in rural areas a thief often has a snack before leaving. What she didn't understand was why the dog had let it happen—although he was quite young. He sat there calmly scratching himself, as if explanations were not in order.

Madame F. checked the house to see what was missing. Everything was there, and she could find no evidence of a break-in. But somebody had gotten in and eaten something; the evidence was there on the kitchen table: the glass, the crust of bread, the jar of preserves. She arrived at the hypothesis that a tramp had come to take a nap and have a meal before resuming his wanderings.

The next day the woman of the house explained the whole thing to her.

"Well," she said, "there is no need for you to dream up a story like that! It was the dog, you see. Without getting caught, he managed to steal some items in the kitchen and place them on the table."

The German shepherd did, in fact, have a habit of taking everything that he could get a hold of and carrying it delicately from one place to another. Thus he was often observed in the garden carefully holding a glass between his teeth. He had never broken a single one!

That particular day, finding himself locked inside and bored, he had decided to set the table!

The only thing is, all dogs are not as intelligent as this German shepherd or my Airedale friend, and it often happens that a glass is broken or that a pin is swallowed during play.

In such a case, the dog must be fed either spears of asparagus or leeks, one after the other. The tips of these vegetables wrap themselves around the object swallowed, envelop it, and thus usher it harmlessly toward the natural orifice through which it will be expelled. This is why I advise my clients with puppies to always keep some cans of asparagus on hand. If you mix them in with chopped meat the dog swallows them readily—and is saved!

In place of these vegetables you can give the dog some very small pieces of cotton mixed in with his meat. But you actually need to have twigs of cotton, or else you risk an intestinal obstruction, which will not help anything!

Hairpins

Coils of hair can be the delight of dogs and the despair of their owners.

I owned a dachshund, and my wife had long hair.

One morning my dog, taking his daily constitutional, as was his privilege, stopped to take a crap (begging your pardon) and then departed. He proceeded for a few steps, wrinkled his brow, resumed his position—nothing. He reflected deeply on this nonevent, did not understand it, resumed his walk, and several yards farther on undertook the preliminaries again, still with no result. He was most embarrassed and I, a young vet, was even more so!

After proceeding for about fifty yards in this fashion, and baffled by my dog's behavior, I examined him guess where, and saw a hairpin protruding. This I extricated as delicately as possible.

The dog certainly had felt something, but it wasn't what he had thought it to be; it was my wife's stickpin, which he had swallowed the preceding evening for his supper. Had I noticed this, I would have given him some asparagus or leeks. Fortunately the sharp end of the pin hadn't perforated an organ.

It should be mentioned that animals in general—not just the ostrich with its celebrated stomach—assimilate the odds and ends that they swallow much more easily than babies do. However, one item can kill them:

Peach stones

A dog eats a peach, including its pit. You might expect that it would make its way to the end of the digestive tract (as is often the case with a pebble); well, that never happens!

The intestine reacts to a rough surface by contracting and

closing around the object; this leads to a fatal intestinal obstruction. So an object with a smooth surface—a needle or piece of glass—can slip through, but something with a rough surface cannot. If this problem occurs, there are two solutions:

(1) to give the dog a purgative (see *Constipation,* page 41) and hope that everything passes out all right:

(2) if the pit doesn't come out, immediately take the animal to a vet for surgery.

Hooks

I was with friends in Touraine whose property is crossed by a branch of the Loire. The weather was fine and we decided to take a boat trip. Just as we shoved off, Adrien, a basset hound, joined our party.

He frolicked about excitedly toward the prow and then, unable to contain himself any longer, suddenly threw himself into the water. Unfortunately, we had on board all the tackle necessary for salmon fishing. I don't know how this clumsy dog managed to do it, but in jumping out he caught a big fishhook in his thigh. The other paraphernalia followed—line and rod—but this didn't stop him from swimming happily to the opposite bank.

There, while his master held him, I operated.

The hook was embedded well into the thigh, and it was stuck there.

Simply to yank it toward me would have been a mistake: I would have torn the animal's muscles and butchered him horribly, without accomplishing anything. I had only a pocket knife for a lancet, but it was adequate. I cut the dog's skin at the spot where the point of the hook was (without doing much harm to Adrien who, being a dog, had much less delicate nerves than a man); then I worked the hook toward that exit point. When it came into view, I cut off the little barbs at the end with a pair of wire cutters that I had found in the boat. I was then able to withdraw the hook without tearing the animal's muscles.

If a similar accident ever happens when you are present, do just as I did.

NOTE: Never try to pull out a hook without having first cut off the end.

HEART ATTACK

Finette and her mistress were only two months apart in age: seven years. Finette, the older of the pair, was a dachshund descended from a dog pack that had spread terror among the gentle foxes of northern France. A granddaughter of the pack leader, she was aware of her high rank and was haughty to the ends of her twisted paws which were so adept at digging into the entrances of burrows so that she could work her way in. She regarded with scorn and condescension all these greyhound-like dachshunds raised as parlor dogs who would have been incapable of overcoming Renard in his den, and still less of diving into the water to the bottom in order to retrieve a wounded teal.

Her mistress was herself the granddaughter of old Wiking, who had owned the pack, doubtless the last in the area.

Finette obligingly submitted to all the fantasies of the little girl whom she loved. In the role of a live doll, she was, by turns, dressed in clothes, tucked into bed, ridden around in a doll's stroller, and deposited inconsiderately in a cupboard. Finette also doubled as a fairyland dog, sometimes even assuming the role of wicked stepmother when the little girl played the princess.

But the role that the little girl preferred over all others was that of doctor.

It happened that her father was the director of a well-known laboratory. He was an austere man in an austere office of serious scholars who came to discuss the most serious matters with him.

To the two little friends, the greatest possible fun was for the great man to go away. When he did, the two of them entered the office on tiptoes—and tip-paws—the little girl carrying some heavy dictionaries, checked out at the library, which she hauled onto her father's magisterial chair and piled up to the right height. Finette then proceeded to seat herself atop the dictionaries with her paws resting in front of her on the desk, as serious-looking as any bureaucrat. To complete the effect, her mistress put a pair of glasses and a beret on her, and stuck a pen between her nails. Outfitted thusly, the dog was capable of remaining immobile for hours in that somber office, while the little girl hid behind a curtain, both of them as patient as could be.

Eventually, some eminent and erudite scholar would appear and say politely

"Good day, Monsieur, how are . . . ?"

And then he would turn a bright red.

The little girl and the dog were never sure if this was from anger or suppressed laughter.

These episodes usually concluded with twin spankings, but these didn't stop them from repeating the stunt. It was just too good a trick!

They tried this game one more time, when an elderly doctor had been left in charge. All at once, Finette abandoned her role and groaned and then reeled to the floor in a faint, still holding her pen in her paw like the person she was imitating.

Crying from fear, the little girl rushed forward from behind the curtain. As for the doctor, he hurried toward the dog and administered cardiac massage, just as for a person. It should be mentioned that he was very fond of the girl and her pet.

After several minutes, Finette came to her senses but she whined softly as if she was hurt all over and in fact she was suffering greatly.

"Is she going to die?" asked her mistress stoically, her face white with anguish.

"No," said the doctor, "but in my opinion she has had a heart attack. We'll take care of her and I certainly hope that we shall save her. Hand me my doctor's bag, will you please? In it you'll find a syringe and some camphorated oil. I'm going to give her a 2-cc injection."

When the little girl's father entered his office, one of the most renowned professors of France was leaning over a little dachshund that he had kept alive so that a little girl wouldn't cry.

Well, here is what you must do if your own dog has heart trouble, which happens to dogs as often as to people.

You can diagnose this serious condition from one of these three symptoms:

(1) A fainting spell like Finette's; these are quite unusual at the first stage. They generally don't occur until the second or third episode.

(2) An attack of pain that paralyzes the dog and that is usually mistaken for a rheumatic attack. In such a case, place your

hand over the animal's heart. The diagnosis isn't certain but it is probable if you either feel the heart beat at an accelerated rate (the normal rate is about 100 beats per minute) or detect an irregular beat.

(3) Coughing spells, usually at night, which give the impression that the animal is trying to spit up something. These are due to edema of the lungs caused by the illness.

In such cases if there is fainting, cardiac massage must be performed immediately (see *Cardiac Massage,* page 81) to revive the dog; "mouth-to-muzzle" resuscitation may even be needed. In any case, in order to ensure that there will be no more fainting, as soon as possible take the animal to the vet, who alone can make an exact diagnosis and administer the proper treatment.

If you are far from a vet, while waiting to see him you can give your pet 2 cc of camphorated oil. Under no circumstances should you give him anything else. And avoid any exertion, any walking, any movement which might aggravate the situation.

LIVER TROUBLE (FALSE)

Being a well brought up dog, Pill, the little darling, asked that someone open the kitchen door quickly. He looked so sick that there was no mistaking it: "He has a liver problem," whispered his mistress.

And in fact, in the corner near the sink, Pill had vomited some bile.

"No food all day," decreed the good mistress, "and this evening you will have a little milk diluted with mineral water."

Miss B. was perfectly correct about the feeding regimen but totally wrong about the diagnosis: dogs never have liver trouble unless they have jaundice. What they frequently vomit in the morning is gastric juice.

When this happens to your pet:

(1) No food all day.

(2) In the evening give him a little milk diluted with mineral water.

(3) If he vomits several times, give him citrate of soda in the recommended dosage. If you have none, give him the following solution, which you can get him to swallow by little teaspoonsful: (See *How to administer a drug*, page 7.)

bicarbonate of soda, *one teaspoonful,*
water, *a small glass,*
the juice of a lemon

DISLOCATED JAW

Bonhomme, the chestnut poodle, yawned; he yawned wide enough to dislocate his jaw—and he did!

He stood there stupified before his owners, his mouth open, without understanding what had happened to him. I had to be called for help. I wasn't surprised because this occurs quite frequently, especially with puppies.

Here is what I did. You can do the same if your dog has the same problem and there is no vet nearby.

(1) I inserted my thumbs into the jaws, one on each side.

(2) I pulled down on the lower jaw as if I were trying to dislocate it further.

(3) I pushed toward the back.

The jaw reassumed its position and Bonhomme graced me with a joyful slurp of the tongue by way of thanks.

DIARRHEA

One Monday a client came to me with her dog, a mongrel whose ancestors had been of the most varied breeds for several generations. His lineage gave him the insolent air of a street urchin. He had a black spot on a white muzzle, and a rakish ear draped on a big nose that was always sniffing around inquisitively. He listened with a blasé look to the words of his mistress. He wasn't at all frightened by my veterinarian's office and tried to strike up a conversation with Romanoff, my blond Afghan who, in such situations, immediately goes into her Grand-duchess of Holy Russia act, that God may protect her from these bastards of revolutionaries!

The mongrel went on with his gentle teasing of Romanoff—or of his mistress, who was explaining to me that since the previous evening he had been having dreadful diarrhea.

"And, of course," she told me, "he hasn't eaten anything that could have made him sick—he has had the same things as we. I made a nice soup and I gave him a big bowl of it—and now look!"

I was looking and beginning to see.

"Were there potatoes in your soup?"

"Of course, Doctor."

"No need to look further; they are responsible for your pet's diarrhea. The starch in potatoes is toxic for dogs, who get enteritis which can even become chronic. That was a veritable detergent that you made your pet swallow when you had him eat those."

His ear cocked to one side, his eyes of jet, the end of his tail like a plume (from what ancestor had he picked that up?), Bastard said to me quite clearly:

"So explain to my kindly mammy that Mama's little bow-wow is a big boy, and as such he likes meat much better than blah-type soups."

I obeyed and explained this, under his watchful eye, while he smacked his lips and contemplated the steak to which my prescription would entitle him. I added to it something that didn't please him quite as much: rice water (a large bowl each day) or limewater (see *Diarrhea in a puppy*, page 74).

So *don't forget:* the potato is a poison to a dog; and there are others.

Noxious foods

These include all the starchy foods—beans, peas, etc.—which can cause fermentation.

Pay attention also to milk. A great many dogs and—contrary to the declarations of the *vox populi*—a fair number of cats don't tolerate milk; this condition is responsible for many cases of diarrhea.

Last and most important, never give a dog poultry or wild fowl bones, which get broken as they pass through the intestinal tract and can perforate the gut (see *Perforation of the Intestine*, page 90). They can also suffocate the animal by blocking the throat (see *Foreign Bodies*, page 43).

The best treatment for diarrhea, if rice water doesn't work, is limewater (see *Diarrhea in a puppy*, page 74).

DYSTOCIA (DIFFICULT DELIVERY)

One of my clients, not very rich and not very bright, dreamed about a toy poodle. Penny by penny he accumulated the sizeable sum needed to buy a purebred dog. His sacrifices were rewarded: he got a very beautiful little dog and, better still, a good pet. He adored her, and she returned his affection. I knew them both very well, for the slightest sneeze made him rush her to me.

By and by he announced to me that he was going to give her away in marriage; the way he expressed it, the betrothal of Miss —— to the Count of ——. He had scrutinized the family tree of her intended from every angle, in order to determine that the male was indeed worthy of his "daughter."

When I heard nothing more about it I thought that everything had worked out well. Then one morning I saw them both, dog and master, coming to my office.

"You know," he announced, "I'm a little disturbed. My Sparrow should be going into labor, this is the time, and I don't see anything happening."

Sparrow wagged her tail briskly. It was obvious that she was feeling fine but that motherhood was the least of her concerns.

"Let's see," I said to him. "When was the honeymoon?"

"Well, it's three months now."

Now a dog normally delivers after two.

I looked at him in bewilderment "Are you sure you're not mistaken?"

"No, Doctor, I couldn't be; I had them marry on my birthday!

That was exactly 92 days ago. So you see, she should have had her babies two days ago."

I had an impossible time trying to get him to realize that his pet wasn't two days late, but 32! He was convinced (like so many other people) that a dog's gestation period is 90 days.

I took an x-ray immediately: the pups were mummified inside the uterus! Sparrow, however, was none the worse for wear.

This can be explained very easily. The uterine environment of the dog is much more closed off than that of a woman; therefore, toxicity cannot occur.

I bring this up to tell you that in a case of dystocia, if you cannot see a vet at once, don't panic. A dog can retain her fetuses for several days without running any risk to herself (see *Delivering Pups,* page 14).

ELONGATION OF A DACHSHUND

With his excessively long backbone supported by four short Louis XV feet, the poor dachshund certainly deserves his various nicknames. But that backbone is also responsible for another thing: the long little dog can easily displace a vertebra or even suffer a herniated disc due to compression of his vertebral column. You can diagnose this when:

(1) The dachshund, a natural comedian, assumes a melancholy air, his tail between his legs and his ears drooping even more than normally.

(2) He can no longer lift himself onto a hassock or climb stairs. There is a very simple way to cure him: do an elongation.

To do so, you need two people. One holds the dachshund in the front, with his thumbs placed behind the shoulder blades. The other holds the tail in his hands and they pull together: the first forwards and the second backwards. Two or three cracking sounds are then audible. Very often these are all that is necessary —obviously, in the less serious cases—to put the vertebral column right.

Basset hounds, which can have the same problems, can be treated in the same manner.

In all cases, however, visit a vet after administering this procedure. An x-ray is often advisable.

POISONING

A colleague of mine once experienced a very unfortunate occurrence. He had to go to a farm to take care of some large animal—a cow or a horse, I don't recall what.

Upon arriving, he left his instruments to soak in a very powerful disinfectant which all rural vets employ, quaternary ammonium salts. To ensure proper sterilization, surgical instruments must be left in the solution for half an hour.

So my colleague left the barn where these preparations were underway, and went to chat with the farmer while waiting.

When he returned 30 minutes later, the dog of the house was dying: he had just drunk the solution of ammonium salts. God only knows why he did such a preposterous thing!

Anyway, you can imagine my colleague's anguish; he came to save one animal and was killing another!

The effect of this poison is practically instantaneous since the animal which has imbibed it is seized by respiratory paralysis which leads to death within several minutes.

I don't know if he got around to performing the operation for which he had come, but my colleague did manage to save the dog. Fortunately, being a vet, he had with him the materials he needed, so he gave the following to the animal:

(1) An intravenous injection of a cardiac stimulant.
(2) An injection of a barbiturate.
(3) A gastric lavage.

While administering these treatments with the farmer's aid, my colleague gave the dog artificial respiration and continued to do so until the animal was out of danger.

I don't expect the same accident to befall one of your pets because this was a highly exceptional case, but I recount this incident to emphasize that an animal can always poison itself by drinking, either from curiosity or some eccentricity of taste, some substance which was never intended for him. This is especially likely to occur out in the country. In such an event, don't forget that rapid intervention is the only thing that can save the animal.

Some common poisonings are:

Copper sulfate poisoning

The symptoms are clear-cut: a half hour or so after ingestion, the animal begins to salivate and vomit and has diarrhea.

(1) Give him some milk to drink just as soon as he can be made to swallow it.

(2) Give him injections of physiological saline solution. In all cases of poisoning, it is advisable to give normal saline to rehydrate the animal. (See *Dehydration,* page 141.)

Poisoning with herbicides

Rhames, a large Afghan, chanced one day to find, growing on a garden path, some tender grass, which he munched joyfully.

He might have died from it. Two hours before, the garden path had been treated with herbicides. These generally have a potassium chlorate base, which is a violent poison.

You run two risks with these:

(1) Say you have prepared the solution with which you are going to water the paths in a sprinkling can. You leave for a few seconds and the dog (or cat) takes advantage of your absence. He drinks from the container which, of course, you have forbidden him to touch.

(2) You have taken all possible precautions, you have locked the dog indoors while you watered the weeds, and you return to your house contented. Yes but animals that like to eat grasses will do just what the Afghan did. The grass, having absorbed the potassium chlorate through its roots, will poison such an animal.

If people do think of the first case, they usually ignore the second. Therefore, while the grass is still alive, keep your pets away from the places that you have treated.

If in spite of all the precautions that you have taken some of the poison is ingested, there is only one solution: gastric lavage.

Only a vet can do this. But if it's a Sunday, out in the country, and you can't find a vet right away, try to get the animal to vomit with some ipecac. Unfortunately this doesn't always succeed.

The dosage for a dog is one tablespoon every 15 minutes until vomiting occurs; for a cat, one teaspoon every 5 minutes.

After you've made the animal vomit:

(1) Make him take some limewater (see *Diarrhea in a puppy*, page 74) into which whites of eggs have been beaten (the limewater is a coating for the intestine and the egg whites serve to fix the toxic salts).

(2) Give him some injections of physiological saline (see *Copper sulfate poisoning*, page 59).

(3) Try to get him to eat some charcoal (see *Diarrhea in a puppy*, page 74).

(4) Give him some strong coffee, which is an excellent cardiac stimulant for a dog.

In any event, after this first aid it is absolutely imperative that the animal be seen by a vet. Even if saved, the animal may very well get nephritis, which can kill him.

Poisoning with rat poison

A bell had clanged at the garden gate and two very pleasant men had called, "Exterminate your rats! We're covering all the towns in this area!"

Thereupon, trailed by a dog who was fascinated by this operation, they had spread some red-colored pellets in the loft, the laundry room, the cellar. . . .

This was very interesting stuff, these pellets that they were throwing around. The puppy, who liked corn, thought that this might be something like that, and so he gnawed at one pellet, then a second, then a third.

Fortunately for him, his owner saw this! Cutting short this deadly feast, the man rushed the dog to me.

Rat poison contains a chemical which counteracts the effects of vitamin K, which is involved in normal blood clotting, and so the rat bleeds to death internally, as though he had some type of hemophilia.

That would have been the puppy's fate too, if I hadn't been able to treat him in time. In such cases a person can't do anything by himself; only a vet can stem the effects of the poison. But don't waste any time!

NOTE: The latency period being from several days to several weeks, if you don't catch the animal in the act, he may be poisoned without your being aware of it. However, you can diagnose this condition because suddenly you will notice a red patch on the dog's belly, and then another one next to it, and then the dog's lips will begin to bleed.

Even at this stage a vet can still save the animal.

Don't forget that in any case of poisoning you absolutely never administer oil to the animal. In fact, the oil mixes with the poison and helps it pass through the intestinal barrier and therefore helps it enter the bloodstream more rapidly.

EPILEPSY

The four-year-old beagle with long ears and a very long tail carried himself with perfect British dignity, as was his right as an Englishman. He lacked only a bowler and umbrella, but spiritually he had them. You felt, when he sighed—and he sure did know how to sigh—that, in the large bright study of a Parisian decorator, he was dreaming of London.

The poor beagle—that day when he took his accustomed place beside Miss D. in their little green Triumph, he didn't know what was in store for him. But he certainly did like that little car, doubtless because, like him, it came from England.

Along the way, suddenly a tractor decided to turn at just the instant when the Triumph moved to pass it. Miss D. only had time to swerve sharply to the left. The car wound up in a field.

Happily, no one was dead or even injured. Miss D. got out, on the whole very happy to be done with this frightening experience. However, having lost all his self-possession and buried by the back of the seat which had fallen on him, the beagle trembled like a leaf in the wind, slobbered, and—horror of horrors—the distinguished canine actually, out of terror, made peepee.

A week later, the young woman had forgotten about the accident when she saw her dog begin to shiver, drool, and then be shaken by convulsions; and finally this dog who was propriety personified urinated on the spot, just as he had following the accident.

In panic, she telephoned me and said, "If a dog can be an epileptic, I would say that he is having a fit."

Certainly a dog can have this malady just like a human, and that is exactly what happened to this beagle.

The nervous trauma that he had suffered as a result of his fear during the accident was responsible for it. I gave him an electro-encephalogram. The epileptic foci were clearly evident.

The beagle survived very well despite his epilepsy. I crammed him full of sedatives but, in spite of them, he averaged two attacks a month.

However, physical nervous trauma is not always the origin of these cerebral short circuits. They can also be the sequel of an infectious nervous disease. Furthermore, epilepsy is sometimes congenital.

Lastly, chiggers or harvest mites, those abominable microscopic creatures, can enter through the ears and cause an attack. (See *Chiggers,* page 94.)

If you have an epileptic dog, don't despair. The animal isn't going to die any more than a human would. Once the fit has passed take the dog to a vet, who will give him a sedative. However, during the attack don't touch him, don't move him, don't pet him, because he might bite you unintentionally. Try merely to slide a piece of wood between his teeth so he won't bite his tongue—but watch your hand!

FRACTURE OF THE PAW

If you are too far from a vet to take the dog to him, or if for any other reason it would take several hours to reach him, the first thing to do is to make a splint. To do so, you need to:

(1) Locate the exact spot of the fracture. This isn't very hard to detect, even for a novice: it can be felt under the toe.

(2) Make a splint running the length of the paw, in order to

immobilize the two joints. Take two very straight slats of wood of the same width and length as the paw. If, as often happens in the country, you know a carpenter who lives not far away, ask him to make it.

(3) Place the slat of wood against the undersurface of the paw, padding it with cotton gauze or, if that's not available, clean rags so that the animal isn't injured, and bind it firmly with a bandage.

(4) To do so, take an elastic bandage and wrap it into a V (see *Dressings of Wounds,* page 88), starting at the tip of the paw regardless of the place of the fracture.

A dog's paw is actually very delicate. If the bandage is placed only over the spot of the fracture, several hours later you will find that either on top or underneath, the paw is red and swollen. In order to be tight enough to stay on, such a bandage acts as a tourniquet and cuts off the circulation, whereupon gangrene may set in. That is why it is absolutely necessary to bandage the whole leg: from the tips of the nails to the thigh. This technique also has the advantage of immobilizing the two joints, thereby not allowing the leg to budge.

I would like to mention another thing. Very often the master, not wanting to cause his dog any pain by touching the spot of the fracture, prefers to position the splint lower down. And that just causes the dog more pain!

NOTE: You can administer first aid to the animal yourself only if the lower part of the leg is involved (tarsals, metatarsals, carpals, metacarpals, tibia, radius, cubitus—the bones below the elbow or knee).

FRACTURE OF THE PENIS

This is an ailment with which only the males of the canine species are acquainted.

The dog, curiously enough, has a bone in his penis—a penile bone—which, like all bones, can be broken.

Now although the Pope himself has authorized humans to practice *coitus interruptus,* veterinarians, being wise men also, have made their own, but just the opposite, decree: to separate animals that are coupling can only have bad consequences (see *Balanoposthilitis,* page 34). In the case of the dog, this step frequently results in a fracture—very painful—of the penile bone.

Don't forget that it is a thousand times better to give a dog an abortion (see *Abortion,* page 34), which is a safe procedure, than to risk injuring your dog by interfering in an act of gallantry. Actually, coitus in the dog is very lengthy and the male cannot uncouple until the act is finished. After a short time together, the male and female begin to get bored with each other and indeed wish to have a parting of the ways. But, as you might expect, Nature has found a way to prevent this (animals don't make love for pleasure, but in order to reproduce), by means of a special kind of erection: two bulbs of erectile tissue lock the male's penis in the female's vagina. If a person tries to pull the male off, the animal turns around and this is what breaks the penile bone. And of course only a vet can deal with such a fracture.

DEMODECTIC MANGE (DOGGY ITCH)

Demodex is a microscopic parasite which is an avowed enemy of pets, which appear gigantic to it. Dogs, especially short-haired ones, are particularly susceptible. And you should bear in mind that the underdog always wins the first battle.

He attacks stealthily and by ignoble tactics: he burrows under the skin, sets up his headquarters, and chews off the hair, at the root, of the territory that he has occupied illegally.

Moreover, he has an ally: water. If by chance you bathe the unfortunate dog at this stage, the parasite takes advantage of this opportunity to gallop joyfully about and totally invade the territory that he has begun to occupy.

For a very long time demodectic mange was not treatable. Today, however, a preparation exists which seems to defeat the parasite. But like all modern medicines it is very dangerous and can be employed only by specialists: in this case, veterinarians.

In the meantime you yourself can temporarily suppress the *Demodex*—although it won't disappear completely—in the following manner:

(1) Have your dog bask in the sun. If you have a sunlamp, you can tan yourselves together in its light, which is also salutary.

(2) Go to your druggist and ask him to prepare you a solution of:

chaulmoogra oil: 75 grams
ether: 25 grams
carbolic acid: 2 grams.

In early times chaulmoogra oil was used to treat lepers. Since very few lepers remain in our country, the druggist doubtless will tell you that this famous oil no longer is available. But be persistent: he is supposed to supply you with it, and it is found listed in his index (but I warn you: it smells horrible!). Apply this solution to the affected areas.

(3) Then wash the animal with a solution of equal parts of ether and alcohol.

In any event, when your dog reaches two years old, the mange will disappear all at once—but it will reappear when he reaches 12 years and will last until the end of his life.

Why? Because the skin of a dog between 2 and 12 years is too tough to be attacked by *Demodex*. What happens to the parasite during this ten-year period, however, remains a mystery.

GASTRITIS

See *Liver Trouble* (*False*), page 52.

ANAL GLANDS

It was the age described in mythology, when the Greek gods involved themselves in earthly matters, and animals spoke. . . .

During that long ago time, a canine congress assembled, for the purpose of framing a constitution for that species. Delegates came from around the world. The Saluki came from the Moroccan deserts to meet with his long-haired cousin from the Afghan steppes. The pompous, enigmatic chow arrived from distant

China. The German shepherd boasted of his consanguinity with Master Wolf and tried thereby to impose his demands. The boxers, the Irish setters, the Dobermans, very much impressed by him, would have acceded gladly, but the fox terriers, the bassets, and the poodles walking between their legs scoffed and wouldn't hear of it.

The president of the convention, a very old mastiff weighing 175 pounds, growled that it would be best to establish a republic in which each dog would have a place.

This idea was much acclaimed, and the dogs voted for it.

But a republic could not be established without authorization from Zeus. So it was decided to send him an ambassador to conduct these delicate negotiations.

For this assignment the fleet-footed greyhound was elected.

"Go and find Zeus on Mount Olympus," said President Mastiff, "and give him this message from me."

"But where shall I carry it?" asked the greyhound, who wasn't as bright as he was fast. "I haven't any pockets."

"You have a natural pocket," snickered an astute little mongrel.

And he slid the official document into the dog's anus.

The greyhound sped off as fast as the famous warrior of Marathon. He laid the message at the feet of Zeus, who read it and wrote out a reply to be sent back to President Mastiff.

The greyhound deposited Zeus's message in the same place where he had put the preceding one and set out toward the dogs who awaited him anxiously.

But the greyhound never reached Sparta where the other dogs were assembled. Legend has it that he died by drowning in the rough Eurotas, but that he managed to pass Zeus's answer to one of his compatriots.

And that is why, ever since, when a dog meets another dog, he sniffs under the other's tail: he is looking to see if Zeus's message is there!

The veterinary facts are not perfectly parallel. Like all other carnivores, the dog has two glands located near the anus which produce a malodorous substance (at least to man). Dogs and humans are not at all in agreement concerning perfumes (ask your pet what he thinks of cologne). These are odoriferous glands which are the object of other bow-wows' inquisitive sniffing. The dialogue exchanged by two such dogs must resemble that of two society people: "Do you always use Chanel No. 5?" "What about you; is that a new fragrance?"

In wild animals, these odors also have a defensive purpose. This is true of the skunk, a charming animal with silken fur, black striped with white, which women admire for the marvelous coats made from it.

But the skunk himself doesn't relish being turned into a fur. So when he sees a hunter approach, he lifts his tail like a plume and squirts out the stinking liquid contained in these glands, in order to repel his enemies by asphyxiating them. Dogs and cats, being much too civilized, don't avail themselves of this defensive tactic, but at certain times, especially in the spring, their glands become engorged and they disseminate this disagreeable odor. If the orifice through which the liquid is released gets stopped up, an abscess is formed which markedly resembles hemorrhoids.

You will first notice that these glands are swollen when the dog (more than the cat) "smells bad." Then, since he is uncomfortable, he rubs his rear end along the ground.

When you see your pet doing this, don't just say, "Look at that dog, he thinks he's a sled." Instead, examine his anus and if you see two tender, purple swellings, realize that they will have to be drained. You can do so yourself. And I advise you to drain them every two months as a normal practice. This should be part of the hygiene of any dog, just the way you yourself bathe and brush your teeth. To carry out this procedure:

(1) Place the dog on a table.

(2) Lift the tail way up in order to allow the anus to drain.

(3) Place a large piece of cotton on the anus and, by applying light friction on the exterior, drain the glands.

This isn't difficult. You—and the dog besides—will get used to it very rapidly and you will thus prevent abscesses. If, however, an abscess does form, here is how you should treat it:

So long as the abscess isn't yet formed and there is simply a painful violaceous induration, apply some cold-water compresses to try to resorb it. I emphasize cold water. Be sure not to use warm compresses, which will increase the congestion.

If it isn't resorbed: either the abscess will open by itself, in which case you treat it as any other abscess; or it won't open, and you'll have to take the dog to a vet who will incise it.

NOTE: If you allow an abscess to form several times, the dog will wind up with a tumor. (See *Tumors,* page 108.)

In this case the vet will have to treat the animal. He'll give it injections of a hormone of the sex opposite to that of the animal.

So don't be surprised if your female dog starts thinking she is a male and begins lifting her leg!

HEMORRHOIDS

I am often consulted about "hemorrhoids." This unpleasant affliction actually is the lot of humans alone. Neither the dog nor the cat can have it; but their anal glands, when engorged, give the impression of being hemorrhoids. (See *Anal Glands,* page 64.)

HICCUPS

This is a problem of young dogs. Puppies, like babies, often have the hiccups. They're no more serious in the one than in the other, and they go away by themselves.

If they should last a very long time, give the animal a mild sedative (see *Sedatives,* page 39).

HYGROMA OF THE ELBOW

(See *Hygroma* in Horses, page 217.)

As with the horse, the idea is to prevent it. When a dog is inclined to lie down "like a cow," cover him with several layers of a big blanket.

Certain breeds, especially those used as watchdogs (for example, German shepherd, boxer), are more disposed than others to assuming that . . . bovine position!

PRECONCEIVED IDEAS

This isn't an ailment—except of the human mind that is too sure of itself! But it's responsible for so many illnesses and even deaths of pets that I am anxious to review the most common of such notions here.

I have heard these things so many times in my office:

"Oh, I'm not afraid of anything happening to my mutt. *Only purebred dogs get sick!*" This is just like saying that only royalty can get polio or the flu!

"My dog can't be sick *because I feed him so well.*" That is, "too much," usually. And viral infections preferentially strike obese animals.

"My dog can't be sick *because I give him a clove of garlic every morning.*" Another widespread but completely absurd idea.

"*Nitwits live longer.*" Completely false; the dogs with the greatest longevity are the greyhounds because their hearts—like those of any athlete—beat more slowly. The little nervous dogs—nitwits or not—are those with the shortest lives.

The dog is sick: "*We'll have to get rid of him because he'll pass the disease on to our child.*" False and preposterous. Except for rabies and of course toxoplasmosis (see *Toxoplasmosis,* page 104), no canine disease is transmissible to human beings, either adults or children.

Lastly there is the "garbage can dog" that is fed all sorts of junk by his owner, who is convinced that it is "*good enough for him.*" That might have been true during the time of prehistoric man, when the dog served as a sort of sanitation official. Since then, however, man has evolved considerably, and so has the dog!

I remind you of the *handful of salt* (see *Constipation,* page 41), that "cure-all" which is often responsible for the death of a pet.

INDIGESTION

If a dog has overeaten, he knows enough to treat himself by vomiting. (See *Liver Trouble* (*False*), page 52.)

JAUNDICE

If a dog with jaundice is saved, it's miraculous. But remember one more thing: it's a miracle that takes place only once. The second attack of jaundice is invariably fatal.

The reason is simple.

According to current practice, if a person has infectious hepatitis, the doctor puts him to bed for six weeks, usually without even giving him any medicine. Only total rest—and, preferably, heat—can effect a cure.

Well then, how do you put a dog in its bed for six weeks, and tell it not to budge?

This is precisely why jaundice is fatal to dogs. As soon as the lassitude caused by the disease dissipates a little, the dog begins to run about and tragedy results.

In addition, dogs always get jaundice following typhus (see *Typhus*, page 109) and piroplasmosis due to the bite of a tick (see *Tick Bites*, page 95; and *Piroplasmosis*, page 96), diseases which weaken the animal and predispose him to jaundice.

You can diagnose jaundice in your dog by the following symptoms:

(1) The whites of the eyes become yellow, just as in man.
(2) The eyes are extremely brilliant.
(3) The lips, when you turn them outward, are yellow.

Of course, the dog is generally being treated for the preceding disease and so the vet will detect the jaundice. But, for example, your pet may have gotten better and you may have taken him to the country. In a situation such as this, while you wait to see the vet you should do the following and, moveover, continue to do it throughout the course of medical treatment:

(1) Feed the dog nothing until the vet tells you what to give him. Let the dog have only mineral water, noncarbonated, which is generally salutary in liver disease.

(2) Don't let the dog run all over the house; confine him to a well-heated room.

(3) Only let him outdoors when he has to go, and on these occasions dress him in a dog's cloak, even if he isn't used to it.

These precautions, more than the treatment itself, may allow you to save him.

NURSING

I was in Provençe on vacation. The marshes resounded with the chirping of locusts. The fragrances of thyme, rosemary, and savory wafted toward me like an offering, and a lively little rabbit hopped three times beneath my feet before turning the white spot of his rear end toward me, rather rudely. The sun cast its golden splendor everywhere, and I strode peacefully toward a large red farmhouse where a dog had gone into labor the previous evening and awaited me for a churching visit.

Proudly she showed me her eight pups, who were nursing greedily.

"She hasn't enough milk to nurse that entire family," I said. "I am going to give you a prescription to supplement her lactation."

I began to write when an old woman entered who was still wearing one of those big black hoods of the Provençals of old.

"You there! What are you up to, trying to make this animal sick with your fancy concoctions and getting my granddaughter to squander her money? That dog only needs to be cared for like a woman! You know, your mother—the poor soul—had you during the war, and with the rationing she didn't have much milk. She was only able to get whatever I could bring her. But to look at you now, it's obvious that you didn't lack anything as a baby."

Of course, the grandmother was listened to more than I, but it was my duty to point out—at some risk—that the dog was giving her whole brood only a little milk.

With all due respect I hereby submit this time-honored "formula." It is made up of:

5 grams (⅙ ounce or 77 grains) of fennel seeds,
5 grams of aniseed,
5 grams of cumin seeds,
5 grams of juniper berries.

These are mixed thoroughly and given to the dog. To aid her to swallow this mixture, it is best to crush it in a bowl of raw meat.

STOPPING LACTATION

One day I went to see some friends whose dog, a superb Gordon setter, had just had pups. Unfortunately, this pregnancy was the result of a moral slip that the dog had neglected to mention, and so her owners observed her growing fat without their understanding why. When they did finally realize the reason, it was too late to abort her.

I found them all upset:

"We'll have to kill the pups now that they have been born."

I don't like to massacre innocents; I grimaced at this proposal.

"You have to at least keep one of them for her to nurse."

I examined the dog's mammary glands: they were hard and she suffered visibly.

"We'll have to stop the build-up of milk," I said. "Have you any whiting?"

Rather astonished, they answered, "Yes. . . ."

"Then bring me some, and at the same time give me a bottle of vinegar."

I made a plaster out of the whiting and vinegar, and applied it to the setter's mammary glands.

Lactation was totally stopped 48 hours later.

Don't forget, then: if for any reason the lactation of an animal must be interrupted, here is how to proceed:

(1) Give her a mild purgative of castor oil, paraffin, or, failing these, kitchen oil. Dosage for:

A *large dog:* castor oil: 1 large tablespoon; paraffin: 3 tablespoons; kitchen oil: 6 tablespoons.

A *medium-sized dog:* castor oil: 1 small tablespoon; paraffin: 2 tablespoons; kitchen oil: 4 tablespoons.

A *small dog:* castor oil: to be avoided; paraffin: ½ tablespoon; kitchen oil: 1 tablespoon.

(2) Prepare a plaster by adding whiting to vinegar until a thick cream is obtained.

(3) Apply it to the animal's mammary glands.

(4) Leave the poultice in place for 48 hours but keep it covered with a bandage so the dog doesn't lick it.

You can follow the same procedure when the pups are weaned, so that the mother's mammary glands don't droop. These are always very ugly, and there is no reason why a dog shouldn't benefit from a cosmetic measure! You can also apply a poultice of fresh chopped parsley, which you secure with a bandage in the same manner. This is a very old recipe which was even used in olden days on the breasts of young mothers, so that once they had finished nursing their baby, their breasts would not sag.

You should change the parsley every morning for three or four days, in order to keep it fresh. Then, for about a week, rub camphorated vaseline onto the mammary glands.

AIR SICKNESS

With fur the color of autumn leaves or of a fox, with the most beautiful eyes in the world, and with a gentleness which made her beloved everywhere she went, Clarissa, a German shepherd, came from excellent stock. Courteous and distinguished, she never allowed herself to do anything that would compromise her dignity.

She dreaded only one thing and showed it by a slight recoiling when she spied the cage which signaled it to her: airplane travel. It wasn't the uncomfortable portable kennel to which she objected. She just curled up into a ball and considered herself as well-off as a passenger with a tourist-class seat.

No; she dreaded air sickness, because she had it every time! This took a great deal away from her air of distinction. When she vomited up bile in the narrow space where she was enclosed, it soiled her! When she finally set her paws on solid ground again, she was always so disgusted and irritable that her master, out of pity, spoke to me about it.

"So why make your fine pet suffer so?" I asked. "Simply give her a sedative with a barbiturate base before leaving. It will make her feel good and will put her to sleep. She will make the journey without being affected by it."

He did just that and Clarissa never again feared air travel.

If your dog too has air sickness or, as often happens, car sickness, give him a sedative before leaving. (See *Sedatives*, page 39.)

NOTE: Barbiturates are now available that will make the dog feel comfortable without feeling drowsy.

DISTEMPER

First, there are diseases for which the owners are in no way responsible: toxoplasmosis, pyroplasmosis. . . .

Second, there are diseases for which they are completely responsible because they can prevent them by having their pet vaccinated at the proper time. The best known of these is distempter.

Our British friends discovered this disease, but a French veterinarian, a contemporary of Pasteur, isolated the virus causing it. The development of vaccines followed. This saved the lives of dogs that formerly the disease used to kill off like flies.

It has since been learned that there is not just a single virus, as had been believed, but 18 different ones responsible for 18 forms of the disease, including a herpes virus as well as others. This is why, at about 2½ or 3 months, a puppy should have his first vaccination. He will have a second vaccination at the age of 4 months, and a booster every 3 years.

A puppy gets the disease only if his master has not done his duty and had him vaccinated.

Whichever virus is responsible, the disease always begins in the same manner:

The puppy is drowsy and refuses to eat; his eyes tear, his nose runs, and he seeks dark places. Then he gets diarrhea and his temperature is slightly below 103°F (39.5°C).

Obviously, when you observe these symptoms, it is necessary to see a vet.

But if for any reason whatsoever you can't see him at once, treat the dog as though he had the flu. Keep him warm and calm and in shaded places, giving him only noncarbonated mineral water to drink.

But *don't forget:* This mild syndrome will almost surely be followed by encephalitis and meningitis, and you have very little time in which to act.

The dog owner who has not had his pet vaccinated is already

very culpable. He should not increase his guilt by waiting until the puppy is lost before deciding to see a vet.

PUPPY DISEASES

Constipation in a puppy

Mommy Dog kept licking her puppy's rear end and massaging his stomach with her big black nose. He was constipated. She was very concerned, but what more can a poodle do? Only Mistress would be able to help . . . but people are sometimes dumber than "dumb" animals, and this one didn't notice a thing.

At last all this disturbance in the dogs' basket caught her attention. She observed the situation and declared authoritatively something that Mommy Dog knew as well as she:

"Your puppy is constipated."

She added, "He can't be allowed to go on like that." This made the poodle sigh with exasperation; she had tried to explain the situation 24 hours before—was it her fault if she hadn't been understood?

Mistress put a little rhubarb sauce in a saucer and offered it to the puppy. It was good and sweet. He lapped it up with delight and everything returned to normal!

So when a puppy is constipated:

Give him a generous spoonful of rhubarb sauce.

If he can only nurse, dilute it in a little water so that it has a syrupy consistency and give it to him from a bottle.

However, if this doesn't suffice, carve a little piece of soap into a size convenient for a small suppository and introduce it into his anus. This will produce radical results.

Convulsions in a puppy

These are always due to worms. (See *Worms,* page 113.)

Otitis in a puppy

Around the age of four months the formerly constipated puppy now runs the risk of ear disease, which is accompanied by runny eyes. This condition is not serious; it accompanies the appearance of the adult set of teeth. In this case the mistress detects it easily. She treats the puppy by simply cleansing his ears with a baking soda solution.

Bad breath in a puppy

The little puppy stretched his legs, opened his mouth wide, and yawned. He felt so secure in the big warm hands that held him. . . .

But his master exclaimed, "Whew! The little bugger has eaten some garlic! He stinks!"

No, Puppy hasn't eaten any garlic. If his breath smells, it's because he has worms! That rule always holds.

So if Puppy smells like garlic it's because he is full of ascaris worms. He has so many of them that, spilling over from his intestine, they invade his stomach, from where they give rise to this characteristic odor. In such a case a vermifuge is called for. (See *Worms*, page 113.)

Diarrhea in a puppy

Puppies get diarrhea very easily. Adult dogs get it less often and usually after a bout of liver disease or intestinal poisoning. In these cases, don't let the animal eat for 24 hours but give him some rice water only. The next day give him some rice with a very tiny bit of chopped meat, and some Evian water. This generally suffices, if the temperature is normal. (Evian water is a noncarbonated alkaline mineral water—*Trans.*)

If the diarrhea continues, however, there is a very simple and effective way of stopping it. Give the dog some limewater, the same limewater that is used for poisonings or for burns.

To make this, proceed as follows. At any drugstore, buy slaked lime (it may be referred to as "commercial marble lime"). Mix together:

approx. 1 oz. (25 grams) of slaked lime
approx. 1 qt. (1 liter) of water.
Let stand for 24 hours, shaking it from time to time.

At the end of this period, decant the liquid; that is, the lime will have sunk to the bottom, so pour off the liquid and throw it away.

On top of the remaining lime, pour about 2½ quarts (2½ liters) of noncarbonated mineral water or boiled water.

Mix, then filter.

Give the dog some of it—according to his size, from ¼ to 1 quart per day.

To make him drink it more quickly, you can mix in some milk (if the milk doesn't give him diarrhea; if it does, give him the limewater straight). In any case, replace his drinking water with this limewater, which he will then drink when he gets thirsty.

Actually, as I have already mentioned, lime is an excellent protection for the gastrointestinal tract.

Four times a day add to this treatment a teaspoonful of officinal charcoal if you have some; if not you can easily make some by burning a piece of bread until it is charred.

By the way, you will often see a dog or cat take a piece of charcoal from a fireplace where a wood fire has been burning, and munch it with relish. Leave him alone; it's fine for him.

Lastly, you can supplement this regimen, three times a day, with a teaspoonful (for cats or little dogs) or a tablespoonful (for big dogs) of an apéritif with a Peruvian bark base. I emphasize true Peruvian bark (cinchona) because it is an astringent which counteracts the diarrhea.

EYE AILMENTS

The dog's vision

Exuberant, frisky, and playful, ears flapping and eyes almost laughing, a charming blond cocker spaniel was in my office, trying to think up a trick to play on me.

His owner, however was distraught.

"I have brought Boull to you, Doctor, because he has lost his sight."

At first glance he didn't give that impression. And after examining the dog's lenses and retinae, I was certain that his vision was intact.

"Absolutely not. He has normal eyes."

Boull's mistress was clearly incredulous.

"Doctor, yesterday in the park he didn't see me. He tried to find me—and he went off in the opposite direction!"

"How far away from you was he?"

"Oh, not very far . . . a hundred yards at most."

"And in which direction was the wind blowing?"

She looked at me as though, having given the latitude and longitude, she would be asked the captain's age. She replied sarcastically,

"You know, I forgot to check yesterday."

"Well then, I'll tell you: the wind blew towards you—and that's what prevented him from "seeing" you. If he had come to you, you would have thought that he had seen you. But it is the wind, blowing in the right direction, that carries your scent toward him; actually, he "smells" you. Dogs see very poorly.

"If you are a hundred yards away, with the wind blowing toward you from your dog, it is almost certain that, even if he is in perfect health and has normal lenses, he won't recognize you!

"Moreover, his eyes will change very rapidly. Boull is now six years old, isn't he? Even if his eyes aren't diseased in any way, his eyesight is already beginning to diminish!"

Double cataracts occur frequently by the age of twelve years. You can detect this condition because the dog butts against objects, and his pupils remain dilated even in bright light.

So, take him to the vet immediately! Cataracts can be operated upon in dogs just as they are in people, except that, since a dog can't wear glasses, his vision will remain weak all the same: between about 28 inches (70 centimeters) and about 3 feet 3 inches (3 meters).

As long as he can see at least that well, don't be concerned if he can't see as well as you can; that's normal.

In any case, even if he should lose his sight, as long as he retains his senses of smell and hearing, it isn't so terrible because he'll succeed in getting around all right.

Conjunctivitis

Caring for a dog's eyes is a very delicate business. For instance, in a case of conjunctivitis or of irritation of the eye in humans, the first thing to do is to bathe the eye or apply compresses soaked with camomile. But that is absolutely forbidden for our canine friends.

Actually, the liquid which bathes the dog's eye isn't at all comparable to human tears, and so the dog can't be treated in the same way. The preferred procedure is to dry the runny eye with a little cotton and take the animal to the vet. But if you can't do so right away, have the druggist prepare a solution of 2 percent boric acid, and wash the dog's eye with it.

Don't forget that a simple case of conjunctivitis can be aggravated if you wash the dog's eye or otherwise apply inappropriate treatment.

NOTE: Conjunctivitis can also herald a viral ailment, a liver attack, or a cold.

Thorn in the eye

The rabbit ran so fast that to try to catch him the spaniel took a shortcut right through a sweetbriar.

When he returned to his master in complete confusion, he didn't have the rabbit but he did have a sweetbriar thorn in his eye.

There was only one thing to do, the thorn being visible and superficial: remove it at once with a pair of tweezers.

One problem existed: Bill's master didn't have a pair of tweezers on him; they aren't the sort of item that you take on a hunting trip.

So he put Bill in the car and left quickly for the house.

I said "put" advisedly. Bill's master had taken the precaution of immediately tying his four paws together so that Bill didn't try to remove the thorn from his eye by himself.

Arriving home, the man grasped the end of the thorn between the ends of the tweezers, withdrew the thorn gently so that it didn't break in the lens, and then put some drops of methylene blue in the injured eye. Finally he untied Bill, who was annoyed but no longer risked being blind!

NOTE: This procedure is only useful if the thorn hasn't sunk completely into the pupil. If this should happen, under no circumstances try to extract it yourself; you'll only aggravate the condition. Instead, carry the animal at once to the vet, who will perform a minor operation to withdraw it.

But before going to the vet, immediately disinfect the eye with several drops of methylene blue, and tie up the dog's legs so he doesn't rub his eye or push the little point in any farther.

Scratched eye

The dog and the housecat got along very well, but one day the dog, who was a year old, could think of nothing but playing. The cat had finally had enough of this, after being jolted awake while sleeping contentedly curled up on a big eiderdown. She struck out at her pal. Unfortunately, her claw caught his eye.

Of course it was Sunday, the whole family was in the country, and no one could find a vet.

If this should happen to you, immediately put some drops of methylene blue (which you should always have in your veterinary medicine chest) in the injured eye. This will prevent the scratch from getting infected. And of course get to a vet as soon as possible.

Ulcerated cornea

Whether it's a sequela of a herpes infection or whether it follows a scratch or a thorn, a corneal ulcer can form in your dog's eye. One sad morning you will notice that he has a little hole in his eye. Don't get excited; treat him just as you would a horse—he will recover just as quickly. (See *Ulceration of the Cornea* in the Horse, page 228.)

Dog "wearing glasses"

Several hours after appearing perfectly healthy, the dog suddenly had eczema completely encircling his eyes. They looked just as if they were circled by eyeglasses. This condition is every bit this "spectacular"; nevertheless, there is no need to be too worried. Treat the dog as you would in any other case of eczema.

"Potatoes" in the eye

These famous "potatoes" which can get into the dog's ears (see *"Potatoes" in the ears,* page 45) or get stuck between his toes can also insinuate themselves between the eyeball and the third eyelid. I discuss this third eyelid with reference to the cat (see *The third eyelid,* page 149); you should be familiar with it.

Of course it is hunting dogs with their sagging eyes (you are familiar with the despondent look of a basset, for example) who are the main victims of this condition.

When you see a little barb sticking out of the eye, which now has good reason to appear unhappy, you must:

(1) Grasp the "potato" with a pair of tweezers and remove it—but be very skillful, I hasten to add.

(2) Then wash out the dog's eye with a solution of 2 percent boric acid. (See *Conjunctivitis,* page 77.)

If you don't succeed in removing the potato from the eye, you'll have to call the vet, who will be more skilled at this than you.

INFECTIOUS HEPATITIS

In 1947, the German veterinarian Rubarth observed that certain puppies, although vaccinated against distemper, got sick anyway. But this illness proved to be unrelated to distemper, whose virus Dr. Carré had discovered. This disease was a viral heptatitis, contagious and rapidly progressive. Its symptoms: the eyes are very blue, the dog vomits. He soon becomes comatose; his temperature reaches and even exceeds 104°F (40°C).

Proceed as you would for distemper (see *Distemper,* page 73), but even more expeditiously since the dog can die in several hours.

VENEREAL DISEASES

Sticker's disease

Much more fortunate than man, neither the dog nor the cat risks catching syphilis or even a common case of gonorrhea. These venereal diseases do not exist in animals!

On the other hand, there is a very serious illness—since it is a cancer—which affects the genital organs and is transmissible by coitus: "Sticker's disease."

Until recently it was encountered only in certain countries or certain regions. In France, for example, until the last few years it existed only in the southwest. But with exportation of dogs, it is now found almost everywhere; that's why we must be acutely aware of it.

Obviously, you aren't able to treat it. But you can detect it and if you do, not only should you take the animal to the vet, but *above all* and *before you do anything else,* whether the dog is male or female, prevent all sexual relations with other dogs, or they will be infected also.

Here is the syndrome of Sticker's disease:

In the male: Reddish, slightly bloody draining sores at the end of the penis. When the penis is erect it is completely deformed and resembles a cauliflower (!).

In the female: obviously the condition is less apparent because the polyps are in the interior, but the same persistent bleeding sores will be present. If you should detect them, at times when she is not in heat, have the animal examined at once.

CARDIAC MASSAGE

A young Doberman was brought to me one day to have his ears clipped! Actually this is a cosmetic operation that doesn't present any danger. The animal is put to sleep so as not to suffer, and then we cut the ear, at the spot where it begins to droop, so as to convert it into a very upright little ear which is supposed to enhance his looks.

And so I injected 1 cc of anesthetic into the vein and . . . no more dog—his heart had stopped beating! Immediately I gave him an injection of a cardiac stimulant—nothing!

There was only one thing left to try: cardiac massage. The heart responded weakly, stopped again, began to beat again, stopped again.

This little game with death lasted 25 minutes!

At the end of this period of time the dog was finally out of danger—but he kept his ears intact!

I mention this incident to point out that cardiac massage in an animal can last a very long time before the heart begins to beat normally again. So you mustn't stop after several minutes, believing that the animal is dead.

Moreover it is much easier to practice cardiac massage on an animal than on a man, the latter having a much broader chest. For comparison, examine a dog: his chest takes the form of the keel of a boat. As you press on the thorax, you feel the heartbeat immediately, much more rapidly than on a man. Lastly the technique of massage is easier to execute; the narrow thorax is taken easily between your two hands. You need make only three movements:

(1) Take the animal's thorax between your hands.
(2) Press down.
(3) Release.

Press down . . . release, until the heart resumes beating. A child can do it.

BAD BREATH

A dog can easily "offend."

This doesn't necessarily indicate that he has stomach trouble, or that he has a delicate liver, or that he has a digestive problem. This "bad breath" is inherent in his being a dog. The facts are that almost all of the digestive process in a dog takes place in the stomach, and it lasts quite a long time: from 6 to 12 hours. And the digestive products spill over rather easily from the stomach to the muzzle.

Moreover, certain breeds are more likely than others to smell bad: hunting dogs and dachshunds. However, there is a very simple and effective means of dissipating this truly disagreeable odor. Buy some chlorophyll pills at your drugstore and give them to the animal. The dosages are always the same and have been indicated previously (see *Sedatives,* page 39).

You can also offer the dog a little Vichy water. Since the odor is due to gastric hyperactivity, mineral water will diminish this and, at the same time, dispel the odor released by the digestive process.

NOTE: Don't give him too much mineral water because, by neutralizing the hydrochloric acid present in the stomach to digest meat, the digestive process becomes more laborious.

A second reason exists for bad breath: dental tartar (especially in the boxer, whose teeth tend to overlap). (See *Tartar,* page 102.)

•

EAR AILMENTS

"Daisies" in the ears

An old client of mine who lived in the country phoned me one day with this poetic complaint:

"Doctor, I must see you; my dog has daisies in his ears."

This seemed rather intriguing, so I went over the same evening to see the phenomenon.

The daisies were, in fact, a fungus. The unfortunate animal, who looked as though he had stepped out of a fashion magazine, had had his ears transformed into a mushroom field!

What had happened?

"Well," explained the old woman, "for some time Finaud was whimpering and scratching himself constantly. I realized that something was itching him. So I went and asked my druggist for something to soothe him. He gave me a veterinary preparation for ear inflammations, and I gave it to my dog yesterday evening.

At first it seemed to calm him down, but today, as you see. . . . Do you understand what has happened!"

Yes, I understood very well. This was the result of one of those patent medicines that can be purchased without prescription but which help along the disease as much as the animal.

This one contained antibiotics which had in fact cured the dog of the mild infection that he had caught. But the problem is that an equilibrium exists between the microorganism and the fungus. When all the microorganisms are killed, the delighted fungi take their place and multiply. Exactly this had happened.

So if your dog has an ear infection, there is a very simple way to treat it: a solution of baking soda: 2 tablespoons of baking soda in a ½ quart (about ½ liter) of boiled water.

Wash out the ears with this solution three or four times a day. It is also perfectly suitable for use against fungi.

NOTE: Avoid "veterinary" medicines without first getting your vet's opinion.

Itchy ears

This condition is due to a small parasite which you can see very easily if you look into the ear with a magnifying glass. It occurs in the dog as well as the cat, and even some smaller mammals, such as the rabbit, can get it.

In this disease the ear is filled with a kind of dark maroon wax. The most striking thing is that the animal, especially if it's a cat—a very nervous animal—goes completely crazy. The miserable creature whose eardrum is infested with these *Sarcoptes* mites has fits which resemble those of an epileptic. If this fate should befall your pet, don't panic; examine his ears. If they have the appearance just described, proceed as follows:

(1) Give the animal a mild sedative. (See *Sedatives,* page 39.)

(2) Clean out the ears, twice a day, with iodized glycerin or carbolic (phenolic) glycerin, available at any drugstore. (See also *Epilepsy,* page 60.)

Continue treatment until a cure is effected.

SNAKEBITE

My but they were handsome, this pair of English setters, their silken fur black and white like dominoes.

This was Morocco, and they lived for the hunt. Out in the bush country the hare, the boar, and the partridge multiplied—not to mention the rabbit! Then too, there was the game sought by poachers, which the dogs as well as their master left alone.

One morning they set out joyously, running around excitedly and barking constantly.

At noon the dogs and their master stopped, like good friends, to have a snack.

Suddenly the male fell into a dead set, barking.

"Come on," said the man, holding out a morsel to the other dog. "Leave the partridges alone and have something to eat with us."

A cry of pain answered him. The setter lifted up his muzzle, from which a kind of ribbon hung peculiarly.

The man cursed, seized a stick, and struck the ribbon, which fell to the ground. Then he took the dog, grabbed his knife, and cut the part of the dog's lip where the thing had been attached which now lay on the ground dead, after having tried to inflict death itself.

The dog howled. The female mimicked him. Blood ran onto the man's hand but the dog didn't protest in spite of his suffering, nor did he try to bite or to run away.

Some time later, the man told me:

"I believe that he understood that I had just saved his life."

The "ribbon" had been what in Africa is called a "minute viper." A dog bitten by it is dead within 15 minutes. A man takes a little longer.

Even without serum, there are ways of saving a man; for example, with a double tourniquet. But the dog is almost always bitten on the lip, where a tourniquet cannot be applied. So there is only one way, if serum is not available, to save the animal: to do what my Moroccan friend did. But you must act fast.

Don't forget, if you live in an area where there are snakes always have a snakebite kit on you when you go hunting; it may allow you to save an animal or even a person. I say "on you" because I don't mean in your car, two miles away.

If by accident you don't have any serum and your pet is bitten on the leg:

(1) Apply two tourniquets: one just above the bite, pressing on the vein; and the other higher up, to shut off the artery.

(2) Wash the wound with water or, if that's not available, with urine (urine is nothing more than warm, sterile water), and remove the broken-off fangs if they remain there.

(3) Enlarge the wound with a razor blade or anything else at hand. In these emergencies don't forget that a piece of broken glass works very well as a lancet.

(4) If your mouth is free of sores, suck blood vigorously from the wound, spit it out, then repeat this several times. If there is a settlement nearby, a farm for example, you can accomplish the same thing with the aid of a vacuum cleaner nozzle or a milking machine.

When you have washed the wound and opened it as much as possible, loosen the arterial tourniquet for 30 seconds. Then tighten it again. This causes blood to accumulate between the two tourniquets. Then loosen the venous tourniquet for 30 seconds. The blood that just came in through the artery flows out through the wound. To assist the flow, massage the leg in the direction of the wound, from above downward. Once the venous tourniquet is back in place, again loosen the arterial tourniquet; repeat this several times. In this way you run no risk of letting the poison reach the rest of the dog's body. To the contrary, you cleanse the wound and rid it of poison by means of these washings with blood. To be absolutely sure that all the venom is gone and that the wound is perfectly clean, about a pint of blood (½ liter) has to flow through for a large dog, and half a pint for a small dog—a basset or poodle, for example.

If the animal was bitten on the lip, since any tourniquet above the nose is impossible, make an ample incision in the lip (a hunter always has a knife) and let the blood flow out for a long time. I mean a *long time;* the dog will never lose all his blood! This is the only way to get all of the venom out. Next wash the wound thoroughly with Javelle water (a bleach and disinfectant —*Trans.*)—5 tablespoons in about half a quart (½ liter) of water—and give the dog some strong, sweetened coffee. Of course, he'll have a sore mouth—but at least he'll be alive!

There are no other remedies.

If there is a vet nearby, you may have time to carry the dog to him. I emphasize "carry"—if you let the dog run, the poison will spread through his body even more rapidly.

NOTE: When you buy snakebite serum, make sure you don't try to use it anywhere but locally, because the venom which it counteracts varies according to the species of snake. As I have just indicated, the vipers of Africa, for example, are more danger-ous than those of France. So serum which is an antidote for the venom of vipers in France won't be strong enough in Africa.

INGROWN TOENAIL

The nail of the dewclaw, the fifth toe of the dog, can easily become ingrown. Since the nail is fused to the toe bone (pha-lanx), you need a special forceps, a "guillotine forceps," to slice the nail without crushing or pinching the end of the digit. So this is the vet's department, but take the dog to him right away. Not only is the ingrown toenail very painful but it can get infected and cause an abscess.

LACK OF OXYGEN

A mammal, like a human, may need oxygen, as in a case of asphyxia for example. Don't forget that for a living being, oxygen is as essential as blood.

If you have plenty of time, you can have a tank of oxygen delivered. But what if it's an emergency? Well, ask the nearest garage mechanic to lend you his blowtorch (they all have them for welding). If he likes animals he'll give it to you without hesitation; if not. . . .

But now that you've procured the oxygen, you still have to be able to use it! And it isn't a matter of putting the dog under an oxygen tent; he isn't a human! So what do you do? Well, it's very simple: take a plastic bag, tie it over the dog's head, and stick the oxygen hose into the bag through a hole that you have fashioned in it!

DRESSING OF WOUNDS

Circular bandage

This is made in a circle, as the name indicates. Simply wrap the bandage around the injured spot, making sure that the width remains the same throughout.

Employ this technique for the neck and the torso in particular (in the latter case, use a very large bandage).

Crossed bandage

Since the bandage always comes rolled up:

(1) Begin by holding the bandage so that it unrolls from above.

(2) Make one normal turn.

(3) The next turn should be off at an angle, and come back to the starting point; then make another half turn off in the same direction.

(4) Wind another normal turn; then make another half turn in the same direction.

(5) Make another slanted turn, but this time in the opposite direction from the first, forming an X.

(6) Repeat steps 2 through 5.

When you have finished wrapping the bandage, the next step is to fasten it. To do so:

(1) Leaving a foot or two (½ meter) of free end, cut the bandage off from the roll.

(2) Tear or cut down the middle of the free end.

(3) Tie a knot to prevent this tear from going any farther.

(4) Tie the two free ends around the bandaged part.

When unwrapping the bandage (if it's an elastic bandage), roll it up at the same time. It will thus be ready to be applied again.

You may wish to fasten the dressing with a band-aid, which you can remove later with ether.

Don't forget: the bandage should be perfectly smooth, without any folds.

NOTE: Never tighten a bandage too much or you'll interfere with the circulation. Only an elastic bandage may be tight, obviously because it has the necessary elasticity.

Leg bandage

If your dog has an injury to his leg which requires a tight bandage that won't come loose, the whole leg must be wrapped, including the toes. I explained this when I discussed fractures of the paw: the legs of a dog (like those of the cat) are extremely delicate; a tight bandage at a single point will act as a tourniquet and may lead to gangrene. (See *Fracture of the Paw,* page 61.)

Tail bandage

This is a crossed bandage, the kind that animals remove most easily. To prevent this, there is only one solution:

Get a leather covering (ask a leather worker to make it) to put over the bandage; have it furnished with eyelets and laces to fasten it. The dog will be very annoyed, it's true, but he won't succeed in getting the bandage off.

Alfort bandage

This is a bandage for the body and I defy the most adroit dog or cat to remove it. To make it, you need a strong piece of cloth approximating the animal's size. Then:

(1) Cut a hole in each corner of the cloth.
(2) Stick the animal's legs through the holes.
(3) Bring the edges of the cloth over the dog's back.
(4) Cut into these edges horizontally to make strips about 1 inch (2 centimeters) in width.

(5) Tie each strip on the left to the corresponding one on the right, making sure these are tight enough so the bandage doesn't slip.

(6) Tie the knotted strips again in the vertical direction: the first with the second, the second with the third, etc.

No four-legged animal can extricate himself from this bandage.

The grandmother's bonnet

(1) Anchoring the end of a rolled-up elastic gauze bandage between the ears, wrap the bandage in front of the dog's left ear and under his muzzle.

(2) Come back to the starting point.

(3) Wrap the bandage *behind* the left ear and again under the muzzle.

(4) Come around behind the right ear; your bandage has the form of a reverse figure 8 at this point.

(5) Go under the muzzle again, then bring the bandage back to the starting point between the ears.

(6) Repeat steps 1 through 5.

(7) When the bandage is finished, attach it *behind* the ears. This is the only place that the animal can't reach; otherwise, he'll manage to remove the bandage with his paw.

If the dog does manage to remove it anyway, here is a little trick: remove the bottom and the handle of a plastic pail, then slip it over the dog's head; keep it in place by attaching it to the collar. The dog is furious but is helpless against this kind of helmet.

PERFORATION OF THE INTESTINE

I once knew a Doberman who died at Christmas because his owners offered him a turkey carcass for a Christmas eve revel. They didn't know that by extending him this treat they were going to kill him as surely as if they were slitting his throat but, alas, much more painfully!

Since they were spending the holidays in the country and they couldn't find a vet, the dog was dead by the 26th, his intestine completely perforated by the poultry bones.

I bring up this disquieting example because I really want to put you on your guard. To most people, for some reason, only rabbit bones are dangerous. But I repeat: bones of all poultry and all game birds can be fatal to an animal.

Don't forget it!

If by chance your dog eats some, hurry to a vet (he alone can operate on him to save him) at the first signs.

You can detect these easily:

(1) The dog is seized by vomiting.

(2) He has what we call a "wooden abdomen" which is hard and which, when palpated, causes the dog to yelp with pain.

INJECTIONS

As with people, these are effected by means of a syringe and a needle. For a dog, you need a large, short needle.

(1) Sterilize the syringe and needle by boiling them for five minutes or by soaking them in alcohol at a temperature of about 195°F (90°C) for a minute.

(2) Rub the injection spot with alcohol or some other disinfectant.

(3) Fill the syringe by drawing up the liquid to be injected.

(4) Attach the needle to the syringe but don't touch the shaft or you will contaminate the needle.

(5) Make sure there is no air bubble in the liquid. An air embolus injected into a blood vessel can kill an animal.

(6) With a sharp jab of the hand, stick the needle in.

(7) Inject the medicine by pushing in the plunger gently.

(8) When the drug is in, withdraw the needle with a quick motion and wash the spot with alcohol again.

Intramuscular

To give this type of injection, stick the needle right into a muscle.

Although intramuscular injections are usually given in the buttock in humans, it is much better to avoid this spot in dogs: the sciatic nerve is almost superficial in them, so you run the risk of a serious accident here.

However, at each side of the vertebral column the dog has a large muscle which you can prick without fear.

For all animals I prefer subcutaneous rather than intramuscular injections.

Subcutaneous

Animals respond extremely well to these injections, and they never get abscesses. You can give as many of these as you wish without running any risk. The best place is the skin of the neck, at the exact spot where mother animals grab hold of their babies to carry them. Hold the thick skin in this area in your left hand and simply give the injection with your right.

NOTE: The skin of animals, especially canines, is like leather, so you have to stick the needle in deeply in order to get through.

Intravenous

It is much better to let the vet handle these injections, but in an emergency remember that you can give them yourself. The usual spots are the vein found on the outside of the back leg, on the bottom third of the tibia; and the subcutaneous vein of the front paw. To locate the latter, hold the dog under the armpits and the vein will immediately stand out visibly.

Two people are necessary for an intravenous injection; here is how to proceed:

(1) Your aide takes the dog's thigh (or shoulder) in both hands and squeezes it tightly, thus effecting a tourniquet, above the injection site.

(2) Then take the animal's leg and grasp the joint firmly with your left palm so that it can't budge. Using the same hand, push on the vein with your thumb so that it stands out.

(3) Now, with your right hand, prepare to make the injection. This is accomplished in two steps:

(A) First prick the skin.

(B) Then the needle enters the vein. You will perceive two sensations in the hollow of your hand

(1) A slight resistance: that of the perforated skin.

(2) A sharper sensation which is accompanied by a slight sound: the needle has entered the vein.

(4) Check to make sure the needle is in the vein by drawing out a few drops of blood.

(5) Inject the drug *very* slowly.

(6) When the injection is finished—and above all if the drug is an irritant—draw up two or three more drops of blood (this assures that if any of the drug is left in the syringe, it won't escape under the skin).

(7) Withdraw the needle gently.

INSECT BITES AND STINGS

Bee stings

Dogs have the disquieting habit of catching wasps and bees, which avenge their own deaths by stinging before they die. A dog stung around the glottis may get Quick's edema, which can kill him. This is especially true if he has been nosing about in a wasp nest and the occupants, outraged at such affrontery, attack in force.

You notice this condition immediately: the dog begins to have trouble breathing, and when you open his mouth you will see that his tongue is swollen. In such a case there is only one solution: to give him an injection of Phenergan (promethazine hydrochloride) right away. Phenergan syrup can also be given, but this is much less effective.

The dosage is:

For a cat or a small dog: 1 ampoule or 50 milligrams.
For a medium-sized dog: 2 ampoules of 50 milligrams.
For a large dog: 3 ampoules.

Any druggist can supply these with a prescription.

NOTE: Don't waste time; this is an emergency. If you don't diagnose the condition in time, you'll have to do a tracheotomy. (See *Tracheotomy*, page 106.)

If, as often happens, the wasp sting is at the level of the tongue, the dog will howl and moan a lot, but this doesn't indicate anything serious. Limit your therapy to applying a vinegar compress, if he'll accept it.

Chiggers

These are microscopic arachnids (not insects) which invade the countryside in August and September and show a marked predilection for beans. But beans do not sustain them—the little vampires are interested in blood. Thus they hop aboard the unfortunate host that they have selected for their meals and set up house, and they become encrusted.

The victim is very often your dog. His abdomen will soon be covered with the chiggers, and he'll be lucky if they do not invade his ears, especially if he's a hunting dog. If they do get in his ears, he'll almost go crazy; chiggers can just about cause epileptic fits!

For chigger bites on the abdomen, use an ordinary insecticide or, instead, pure vinegar or Javelle water diluted in an equal volume of water.

NOTE: Never treat a dog's ears in the same manner—that would be catastrophic! Use carbolic glycerin on them, and if this doesn't suffice consult your vet, who will prescribe the same drops (with an insecticide active ingredient) used for demodectic mange.

Flea bites

On the right side of my country home, I have neighbors who are pretty tidy. On the left there is a stud horse.

My house is closed during the winter and when I arrive in the spring, bushels of fleas, coming straight from the right side of my property, alight on my unfortunate dogs.

So I borrow a horse blanket from my neighbor on the left, on which I make my Afghan and basset lie down. The next morning they are rid of all their fleas . . . but they smell like horses.

If you live in a rural area, I recommend this old remedy, unless you prefer to use litter made out of ferns, which is very effective but less so than the blanket.

Of course there are also insecticides—but beware of DDT. (See *Poisoning,* page 57.)

Tick bites

This is a miniscule vampire which burrows into its victim and then fills itself up—its head also—on blood.

The tick (only the female attacks man or other species) is horribly dangerous to dogs because it can transmit a terrible disease to them: piroplasmosis (see *Piroplasmosis,* page 96), which usually results in hepatitis. In one case out of two the dog dies.

If you live in or go to the country, and especially if you hunt, carefully examine your dog every evening. The tick, a mini-Dracula, usually lodges in the throat, but it can also be found in any other part of the body.

NOTE: Don't pull it off; the head will remain in the skin, thus causing a painful cyst. So before killing the tick, you have to make it let go. To do so, let a drop of mineral oil or ether fall on the tick. If you have neither, do as the English do and touch it with the end of a lit cigarette.

Then, one week later, carefully inspect your dog; if he manifests the slightest symptom of jaundice, treat it at once. (See *Jaundice,* page 69.)

Don't forget that his life is in danger!

WOUNDS

Skull wounds

The more a skull wound bleeds, the less serious it is. All you need to do is stop the bleeding with a large gauze pad soaked with hydrogen peroxide, Dalibour water, or, if it's all that's available, chilled boiled water. Then apply a "grandmother's bonnet" elastic bandage. (See *Dressing of Wounds,* page 88.) If the wound is serious, it will have to be sutured also. (See *Suturing*, page 97.)

NOTE: Do not give aspirin, which is an anticoagulant that may increase blood loss. (See *Sedatives*, page 39.)

PLASTERS

Your dog has had a fracture of the paw. The vet applies a plaster and it annoys him; he gnaws at it.

You leave him alone for an hour, and when you return, he takes the opportunity to nibble away at the plaster to such an extent that his toes are now free—to his great satisfaction and your consternation.

However, since the fracture is higher up, you scold him as a matter of principle but you feel that he has done nothing serious.

The next day, to your astonishment, the end of the exposed paw is red and swollen. What has happened to it?

Well, as already explained (see *Fracture of the Paw*, page 61), a wrapping that doesn't run the entire length of the leg will act as a tourniquet. So be sure not to waste any time returning to the vet for a new plaster; otherwise your pet may get gangrene! If you can't see him at once, break the plaster off completely, put on a splint, and apply a bandage along the whole length of the leg.

PIROPLASMOSIS

Ten years ago, when I had moved to Paris, one of my colleagues asked me for some advice.

"I have a dog," he explained, "with an illness that is obviously serious but I haven't been able to diagnose it. Since the dog comes from North Africa, I thought that it might be an exclusively African condition and that therefore you might be better able to make the diagnosis than I."

So I examined the animal, a magnificent brindled Great Dane who certainly looked his 175 pounds (about 80 kilograms). Indeed, I recognized what he had right away: piroplasmosis.

My colleague hadn't been mistaken. I was able to diagnose this very serious illness, which at that time was hardly seen in France, not from having treated it in Morocco but rather in America!

Several years previously while studying in the United States I had, in fact, encountered similar cases several times. And nowadays no Parisian vet would need my help in diagnosing it; they are all familiar with it because, unfortunately, it has spread, first to southwestern France and then throughout the country.

The enormous Great Dane had been laid low, in a battle in which he was actually at a severe disadvantage, by a tiny enemy whose weight hardly exceeds 2 grams: the tick!

This arachnid is *always* responsible for piroplasmosis since it transmits to the dog the microscopic parasites that enter the red blood cells and make them burst. The disease can be fatal if it isn't treated in time. Moreover, it is often followed by jaundice (see *Jaundice*, page 69), which is also very grave.

So beware if your dog has been bitten by a tick. After removing the tick you still have to observe the dog for a good week thereafter, for the incubation period is 8 to 10 days.

The following are the symptoms of piroplasmosis:

The dog is listless and, above all, horribly sad. This sadness in an animal is very curious because it indicates a serious condition.

Then he starts running a fever; generally, his temperature climbs to 104°F (40°C).

When this happens, examine his urine carefully. If it is deep brown like tincture of iodine, there is no mistaking the disease and the dog must be taken to the vet as fast as possible: your pet's life is in danger.

This is true all the more because untreated piroplasmosis almost always leads to jaundice. Piroplasmosis plus jaundice . . . there is little chance that a dog will survive them. Therefore you should make the most of your dog's slim chances: the rapidity with which treatment is initiated is one of the most important factors in curing the disease.

SUTURING

His master was holding a razor blade in his fingers when Farmer, ten months old, felt an urgent need to throw himself at his master's neck to indicate undying love.

Who should be adjudged the clumsier, Farmer or his master who tried to push the dog away? I wouldn't know, but two seconds after this show of affection a bright red slash stretched across the schnauzer's chest. The blade had gone all the way through the skin for a good four inches (10 centimeters). It was very clean, very neat, and very serious—even if sewn up.

As luck would have it, the D. family was out in the country and the mechanic had come that very morning to take the car away in order to change the tires. He wasn't going to bring it back until evening. So it was impossible to get to a vet but it was out of the question to wait patiently until Farmer bled to death. An injury of that extent does not heal by itself.

"All right," Mr. D. said with a sigh. "I'm going to sew you up myself. Fortunately, I have seen the vet do this sort of thing. I can't do it as well as he, but too bad. Go lie down, idiot, and try not to budge!"

Farmer obeyed meekly; he wasn't feeling very proud of himself.

"Bring me your spool of strong thread and a needle," Mr. D. called to his wife, adding, "And bring me the bottle of brandy, too, so I can sterilize them!"

He washed his hands, rinsed them in alcohol and sprinkled some on the wound at the same time, and then dipped the needle and thread in the bottle. Next he began to sew while his wife held the dog, who had no intention of budging anyway.

That evening he brought me the dog, who had been patched up remarkably well, and explained:

"I did it as though my wife had asked me to fix a roast for her: with a double knot. I cut off the thread, I began again at the edge. . . ."

It was perfect; I didn't even have to retouch the job.

If something like this happens to your dog, here is how to proceed as Mr. D. did.

(1) Wash your hands with soap and water, then rinse them in alcohol to sterilize them.

(2) Take a sewing needle and linen thread, if possible, or better yet, nylon fishing line.

(3) Soak the threaded needle for five minutes in alcohol at 194°F (90°C), or else in anything that contains alcohol: brandy, etc.

(4) While this is going on, clean and disinfect the wound. (See *Wounds,* page 95.)

(5) Bring the two edges of the wound together with the aid of a pair of tweezers that you sterilized along with the needle. Don't let the edges overlap, however.

(6) Make a stitch to bring the edges as close together as possible, and tie a surgical knot. To do so:

(A) Make a double knot; that is, stick the thread through the knot twice in a row.

(B) Take the two ends of the thread and tie another knot in the opposite direction; that is, if you passed the thread from right to left to make the first knot, this time pass it from left to right.

(C) Finish up with an extra knot made in the same direction as the first.

(7) Eight hours later, cut the threads and pull them out with a pair of tweezers sterilized with alcohol.

If by chance you have neither thread nor needle (or simply lack the nerve) but do have insulating tape or band-aids, you can secure the edges of the wound together after having juxtaposed them by applying the tape or band-aid.

Then apply a bandage that holds well, or else the dog won't be satisfied until he has pulled off the whole thing.

Usually the dog—especially if he's big—will let you operate in peace. But if you have a nervous animal—a cat, for example— your "assistant" will have difficulty holding him down. If so, "anesthetize" the animal by making him drink a small glass of alcohol. He will be "dead drunk" and you'll be able to operate at your ease.

RABIES

Several years ago on Réunion Island there was an epidemic of bovine rabies. All the steers and cows were attacked by this terrible disease, one by one. Where had it come from? What were the carriers? Naturally the dogs were accused; will they be blamed for this scourge eternally? But the fact was that not a single dog on the island had rabies!

The cows, on the other hand, continued to die. The greatest precautions—separating animals from each other—were to no avail; nothing seemed to work. Several miles away, in areas which hadn't yet been contaminated, suddenly a cow was found to be affected. So there had to be some other animal which was also affected, one that wandered around without fear of traveling freely.

The cattle raisers stood guard 24 hours a day watching for this werewolf who, lurking in the shadows diabolically, marked the herd for death.

They saw nothing.

However one night, while all the cattle were sleeping peacefully, one of the men spied a vampire stuck to the neck of a steer. But don't scream about Dracula; the "vampire" was only an immense bat with a wingspan of easily 4½ feet (1½ meters). It lived on blood, of course. These vampire bats are numerous on Réunion Island, and no one pays them any more attention than we do our owls. The bat dined tranquilly; its meal didn't awaken. However, the man had noticed the steer that it had bitten. Suddenly growing suspicious, he separated that steer from the others. And several weeks later, rabies showed itself in that animal.

So it was the bats that had rabies—a regular horror film! And the dogs didn't have it because, being light sleepers and not wanting to be treated as steak, whenever a bat approached them they protected themselves; they were never bitten!

I have related this story worthy of Hitchcock in order to emphasize that all mammals can get rabies and so can transmit it.

In truth, people often are inclined to forget or to ignore certain essential precautions, especially when out in the country. A dog viciously bites someone; subsequently the dog is killed with a pistol or a stick—without waiting for the vet! A dog felled by a bullet to the head renders any diagnosis of rabies impossible. There is only one course open in such cases: just to make sure, the person bitten is given the very painful anti-rabies treatment of 21 injections in the abdomen.

Rabies is the only disease recognized by the law as contagious for people. Therefore I take this occasion to remind you of what the law requires.

If a person is bitten by a dog or a cat which is suspected of having rabies:

(1) The animal should *never be killed* but instead taken to a vet, who will keep it under observation for 15 days. If rabies manifests itself in the animal, the bitten person must immediately undergo anti-rabies treatment. The animal's saliva can transmit the disease 10 days before the appearance of the first symptom.

(2) If the animal dies or disappears (a wild dog may attack and then flee), the bitten person should be given anti-rabies treatment.

NOTE: Don't mistake an epileptic animal for one with rabies. But don't assume the contrary attitude either, of "not believing in it." Rabies still exists, especially in Eastern countries.

Several months ago, one of my clients brought a puppy back from Germany. One morning she noticed that the little animal was having trouble swallowing. Thinking that he had swallowed something while playing, she felt around with her fingers in his throat and, finding nothing, finally brought the dog to me.

The dog had rabies. Difficulty in swallowing is one of the first symptoms of it. I had to give him an injection and my client, even though she had not been bitten, had to have anti-rabies treatments. The saliva of a rabid animal transmits rabies, even if the person is not bitten. *Don't forget this.*

PREPUCIAL SECRETIONS

People often bring a young dog to me and say:

"Doctor, he has some pus . . . there."

This prudish "there" refers to the dog's penis.

However, this isn't pus, it's a physiological secretion which is perfectly normal in dogs. It is present when the dog gets to be about seven months old. He begins to reach maturity then, and it's a prepucial secretion which his alarmed master mistakes for pus.

As a rule, nothing needs to be done. Dogs make their toilet very capably, without requiring help from anyone.

However, if the secretion is too abundant, the penis should be cleaned with Dalibour water or, instead, with a solution of alum: 10 grams per quart (liter) of boiled water. (See also *Balanoposthilitis,* page 34.)

TARTAR

(See also *Bad Breath,* page 82.)

The handsome Dalmatian, whose coat looked something like mourning clothes, wasn't even seven years old when he lost all his teeth!

His mistress brought him to me but it was too late. The dog had advanced alveolar pyorrhea and I couldn't do anything for him.

"What do you give him to eat?" I asked Madame C.

"Oh, nothing but chopped meat with some rice and grated carrots."

"Never any bones?"

"Never!" she retorted indignantly.

"Well, since your dog hasn't had to do much chewing, he has gotten the disease of overcivilized dogs. Hasn't it ever occurred to you to clean his teeth?"

She blushed with shame.

"My word . . . I didn't know . . . should I have?"

"Yes, actually, since he wasn't able to clean them himself on a bone, or by gnawing on a piece of meat (see *Bad Breath* in cats, page 152). As a result tartar collected on his gums and teeth and worked away at the necks of his teeth, causing him to loose them."

This can be simply prevented, however. Every day, or every other day, quarter a lemon and rub the dog's teeth with it. Lemon converts calcium tartrate into a soluble citrate; in other words, it breaks up the tartar. If you wash your dog's teeth with lemon regularly, no tartar will be deposited and alveolar pyorrhea will thus be prevented.

Furthermore, don't be afraid to give him a large beef bone or, better yet, a veal bone, once a week, on which he can "exercise his teeth."

This can never be overemphasized: check very carefully for these tartar deposits which:

(1) give bad breath;

(2) work away at the necks of the teeth and begin to undermine them;

(3) are often responsible for dental abscesses. (See *Dental Abscess,* page 10.)

TEMPERATURE

I can no longer keep track of the number of clients who have telephoned me to say, "Doctor, my dog has a fever: the muzzle is all warm."

Well, this popular belief is absolutely false. It isn't necessarily true that if your faithful companion has a warm nose, or even a slightly dry one, a high temperature also exists. Perhaps the animal simply slept near the fire or something like that.

The normal temperature of a dog varies between 100.4 and 102.2°F (38 to 39°C); anything above this constitutes a fever. But you can only determine this by taking his temperature. To do so:

(1) So that the dog at least will be in a good position, set him on a table. That will be easier for you and, being disoriented, he will be less resistant.

(2) Lift up the tail and stick the thermometer into the anus *above* the mercury; that is, stick part of the thermometer, where the gradations are, right in.

NOTE: Don't take your dog's temperature by putting the thermometer in his mouth—he'll break it—or under his armpit—that won't accomplish anything!

Furthermore, temperature is a bizarre phenomenon in dogs and is never a good medical indicator; it is too variable.

I recall a charming black poodle that his master brought to me for some benign condition—to have his nails cut, I believe.

I took his temperature routinely . . . surprise—it was 105.8°F (41°C)! I examined him with my stethoscope; I checked his heart, his lungs . . . I found nothing. Just to make sure, I gave him an antibiotic and asked to have him brought back to me the next day.

The next day: the same temperature. For three days I gave him antibiotics, without getting his temperature down.

The fourth day I had an idea. I asked his master to take his temperature at home—and it was 101.3°F (38.5°C)!

The excitement of being in my office had caused his temperature to rise by that much!

This happens quite often in the small, nervous, easily frightened breeds.

TETANUS

Dogs can get tetanus just like people and horses. The only difference is that dogs don't die of it!

A dog with tetanus has very erect ears, a very erect tail, and . . . he "smiles."

Immediately give him a sedative or a euphoriant in the dosage that I have indicated (see *Sedatives*, page 39). But above all, take him to the vet right away; he alone will know how to care for the animal, but without giving him an injection of tetanus antitoxin, for that doesn't accomplish anything.

Don't worry; the dog will be saved.

TOXOPLASMOSIS

I was in Berlin visiting a German colleague when someone brought him a giant schnauzer, a magnificent animal that seemed in no way ailing.

"I don't know what's wrong with him," said his master, "but he isn't the way he usually is."

"Is he eating all right?"

"He's eating fine."

"Is he drinking? Does he sleep?"

"Yes."

"His stools? His urine?"

"Perfect."

My colleague and I exchanged a glance of amusement. It wasn't the dog, but the master, that seemed to "have something."

But to satisfy his conscience, *Herr Doktor* took the dog's temperature anyway: 104°F (40°C). . . .

We exchanged another look, but this time one of astonishment. Well, well! Maybe the owner was right after all! A pet is a little like a child: the "father" or the "mother" is aware of an illness almost before it shows itself, and the doctor who makes fun of the parent is often wrong!

So my colleague gave the dog a penicillin injection as a general precautionary measure and asked to be kept posted.

Three days passed and then a phone call came from the schnauzer's master: whenever someone petted the animal, he groaned as though he were being hurt.

"He must be having an attack of rheumatism," my colleague said to me. "But I have some emergency cases which concern me more than he. Would you be kind enough to visit him and give him a cortisone injection?"

So I picked up a box of the drug at the veterinary pharmacy and went to give the schnauzer an injection.

Alas, that evening, I realized that, being poor at German and having been fooled by a similar package, I had given the wrong drug; instead of using cortisone, I had employed a sulfonamide intended for treating a disease which is rare in France: toxoplasmosis. Anyway, this error wouldn't prove dangerous to the animal; I simply had to give him another injection.

But the next day, there came a telephone call from the owner vindicating me: the dog seemed cured!

"What did you do, anyhow?" asked my Berlin colleague, slightly vexed at the success of a Parisian.

And so I confessed my mistake to him, a mistake which, because of this happy result, permitted us to make an exact diagnosis: if the dog got better, he must have had the disease for which—without knowing it—I had treated him.

It should be noted that toxoplasmosis exhibits a peculiarity: nothing betrays it! Its only symptom: no symptoms! This renders diagnosis rather difficult.

Everything was turning out for the best when I saw my colleague turn pale and pick up his telephone to call back his client:

"Tell me, your wife isn't pregnant by any chance? Yes? All right, I would like you to bring your dog back to me and allow me to keep him for a few weeks, by which time all danger of infection will have passed. I would also like you to have your wife examined by a physician, in order to be sure that the dog hasn't contaminated her."

He hung up the phone. "Let's hope that there aren't any serious consequences," he said with concern.

And since I looked at him in astonishment, he added:

"Here in Germany we think—note that I say 'we think,' because there is no clinical proof of this—that toxoplasmosis is, along with rabies, of course, a disease of dogs which is transmissible to humans. And we 'suppose' that if the person affected is a pregnant woman, this can have very serious repercussions for the fetus."

I have recounted this incident only in order to lead to this conclusion. Toxoplasmosis is a little-known disease whose diagnosis is difficult to establish and which my German colleagues "think" can, if transmitted to a pregnant woman, lead to congenital malformations.

This isn't a certainty, it's an opinion. It could be true, however. So it is better to take precautions, even if they prove to be unnecessary, than to risk a tragedy.

Moreover, since September, 1972, women doctors have drawn our attention to this disease. At a convention held in Paris, they likened the danger of toxoplasmosis (which can, incidentally, be contracted in entirely different ways) in pregnant women to that of German measles. The latter, of course, has possibly dangerous consequences for the fetus. . . .

TRACHEOTOMY

I have told you the story of Youka who, having had a goose bone in her throat, was saved *in extremis* by her mistress. Things don't always turn out so well.

One evening I was dining in the country with some friends. It was a peaceful August night heavy with the scent of honeysuckle.

Out in the garden a chow of eight months played with a stick under the fond eye of her owner, Pierre.

The arrival of this round, tawny face six months before had changed the man's life. He had trembled with excitement like a child when his wife had given him the dog for Christmas. Tio's black tongue had caressed Pierre's hand, and it was as though they were pledged to each other for life. From then on they were inseparable.

When a man and a dog fall in love with each other in this way, they establish an understanding between them that makes women jealous. Their camaraderie is that of two lads: a perfect understanding which has no need of words in order to be conveyed.

I remember well the words of one of my friends who was mourning, with tears, the loss of his Belgian sheepdog who had just died:

"He was my pal . . . every morning we went to take a leak together. . . ."

You have to be a man and to have had a dog to understand.

Suddenly Pierre remarked, "That's funny, I don't hear Tio anymore."

"He has played all day," I said peremptorily; "he's asleep. You know, at eight months he's still a puppy."

I sensed that he was worried and I smiled to myself. Neither his wife nor I, convinced as we were that I was correct, felt like getting up to see what the chow was up to. However we should have been suspicious. Little dogs, like little people, are sophomoric: they do foolish things.

Unable to contain himself any longer, Pierre left the table:

"I know that I'm being ridiculous, but I'm going to see what he's doing."

Paying no attention to his apprehension, his wife continued speaking to me. A cry of anguish made us jump:

"Jean, come quickly . . . Tio is dying!"

We hurried over. Pierre held the chow in his arms; all that remained of his vital energies—very little, I saw at once—were concentrated in the expression of supplication that he turned toward his master. With white foam around his mouth, Tio suffered. I remembered the stick with which he had been playing all afternoon; doubtless a piece of it had broken off and was stuck in his throat. I opened his muzzle. I probed with my finger: his throat was completely blocked by edema. The flesh which was swollen around the foreign object prevented all passage of air. There was no time to try to remove the fragment of wood. The dog had to be allowed to breathe—which called for this procedure:

"I am going to give him a tracheotomy."

I always keep a trocar in my medical bag. I thrust it through the skin around the tracheal artery; immediately the air passed through the big needle and went directly to the dog's lungs; his eyes opened up, and I felt his heart begin to beat again. He was saved and I was able, without fear of having him die, to disengage the piece of wood which was wedged in his throat.

The same thing can happen to you. If so, do what I did, without hesitation. Since the dog is lost otherwise, you don't risk anything by acting boldly. Lastly, performing a tracheotomy on an animal is the easiest thing in the world:

(1) Obtain a trocar (a very big needle; it's a good idea to keep one in your medicine cabinet).

(2) Locate the tracheal artery—there's no mistaking it, you can feel it under your finger.

(3) Plunge the needle in with a firm motion; this suffices to allow the air to pass.

Once you've removed the cause of the respiratory difficulty the hole should be repaired. As this was an emergency procedure, though, you should call a vet for further instructions.

TUMORS

Tumors are distinguished from abscesses by two properties:

(1) They are not warm to the touch, except for expanding tumors.

(2) Their surface is dented (a little like a pineapple).

The most classic tumor is:

Tumor of the mammary gland

This generally appears two months after the hunting season
and is due to a burst of nervous lactation. The tumor becomes
violaceous and painful, so rapidly that this can occur in the space
of a weekend. But if you are far from a vet, you needn't worry;
don't touch it, it will open by itself. When it does, disinfect the
sore like an ordinary abscess, with the aid of an astringent solution (see *Abscess* in Cats, page 122). Then apply a small albu-
plast bandage.

NOTE: What has just been described constitutes first aid. Subsequently, and as soon as possible, take the animal to a vet.

TYPHUS

Disease of Stuttgart

In that shameful year of 1968 a population of two million
individuals was seized by panic: every source of food was going to
be exhausted; it was total, abject poverty. For families used to
eating, and used to eating well, the news was catastrophic. Each
of them became aware of how it must feel to live in an under-
developed country.

Nevertheless this was the fate which was about to befall the
rats of Les Halles when the city council of Paris decided to
transport their natural larder to Rungis instead!

But how did these voracious and clever fellows, whose intelligence is so acute that it has been compared to man's, get wind of
this project? Did they know that the ordinances were signed
which would take the bread and bacon from their mouths, not to
mention the tender rosy carrots, the tart-smelling cauliflower, the
crisp radishes? Nobody knows how they did, but they knew
about it!

There then took place, in the lower reaches where this secret
population dwells, a mobilization for combat.

You may recall World War II and its restrictions. Did this new
mobilization not call for sacrifices, on the part of the female rats,
which were worthy of the matrons of old? The "mamas" had

decided that in place of six litters of six rats per year, they would have only two of two pups—so long as conditions lasted as they were. Thus the offspring could continue to be amply nourished despite the restrictions. This was accomplished without the aid of pills or other human abominations simply because these heroines had decided to do so!

These ladies kept their word for the four years of the war. But as soon as it was over and the ration cards were thrown in the wastebasket, they quickly resumed their customary rate of 36 babies per year! It's true that up to this very day, man has not yet succeeded in explaining this phenomenon. In order to solve the problem, it must be admitted that the rat has a biological intelligence. It is unfortunate that, in this respect, man is inferior to the rat; otherwise we would have no worries about the year 2000! (Actually, many mammalian species appear to regulate their reproductive rates hormonally under stressful conditions such as crowding or starvation—*Trans.*)

This time, however, the situation was much more serious: it wasn't a matter of rationing but of the total disappearance of food.

So the decision was made: like the children of Israel leaving Egypt for the Promised Land, the rat population in its entirety decided to follow its food source and migrate to Rungis.

Two million rats left Paris!

Grandfather, grandmother, papa, mama, and the children packed up, said adieu—one can imagine the tears in their eyes— to the sewers and the cellars that preceding generations had inhabited for more than one hundred years, and the great exodus began.

If Parisians weren't aware of it, that's because the grey population of the night, accustomed to living in secrecy, traveled only during the hours when people are usually asleep.

However, you are correct in thinking that two million rodents wouldn't travel for 20 miles without having to satisfy their natural needs. Our heroes, therefore, relieved themselves along the way whenever the necessity arose.

The following day the bow-wows, taking their morning promenades, breathed in these unusual and very interesting fragrances —and an epidemic of typhus broke out among all the dogs of Paris! For the rat, who himself never has typhus, is a perennial carrier of typhus germs. By inhaling the strong odors that rats leave behind them, the unfortunate dog takes in the virus of this terrible disease at the same time.

Thus each epidemic is almost always preceded by a migration of rats. Even in ordinary times, isolated cases occur which amount to quite a good number per year.

That is why, when you have your puppy vaccinated against distemper, have him vaccinated against typhus too.

If you don't do so and thus fail in your responsibility, here are the symptoms which will allow you to detect the disease.

The dog is apathetic, sad, and refuses to eat.

Almost immediately he is seized by hemorrhagic vomiting and diarrhea; you might say that the animal empties himself of his blood by these two routes at the same time.

In 48 hours the level of urea rises to 3 grams, the kidneys are blocked, and it is the end.

Typhus is thus an emergency; it's not a matter of waiting until the weekend is over to care for the animal! Moreover, any vet will have you come over at once, or will call on you, if you describe the symptoms of typhus to him.

If he is far from your house, or if you cannot meet him immediately, while waiting, give the dog:

(1) an antinauseant. (See *Vomiting*, page 115 and *Internal hemorrhage* in Cats, page 135.)

(2) An intestinal hemostatic by mouth or preferably by injection (see *Injections*, page 91).

(3) Some vitamin K, which any pharmacy can supply without a prescription.

(4) Injections of physiological saline (see *Malnutrition* in Cats, page 139).

HIVES

When he was brought to me, the dachshund resembled a bull terrier: he was swollen everywhere, to the point that you couldn't even see his eyes.

"This dog has been in bad company. Has he, by any chance, been playing with some processional caterpillars?"

His master looked at me the way Dr. Watson regards Sherlock Holmes.

"How did you know?" he exclaimed. "We have had an invasion of caterpillars in the area. They have invaded all the fruit growers' properties; it's a disaster, we won't have a single cherry this year."

"Anyway, as for my dachshund, he has a giant urticaria given to him by these caterpillar damsels whom he is sure to have investigated."

Are you familiar with these "processionals"? They are those charming furry caterpillars. These creatures produce an extremely irritating toxin to which short-haired dogs are highly allergic: dachshund, boxer, French pointer, etc. This allergic urticaria is much worse than urticaria due to alimentary intoxication.

In the absence of caterpillars, nettles can also be responsible for it. For some unknown reason, only short-haired dogs are susceptible; long-haired dogs are insensitive or only slightly allergic. So a dog like the basset, for example, doesn't even have to roll on the nettles—he may have merely sniffed them—for the allergy to break out immediately. It generally begins on the muzzle and the tongue, which have been in contact with these poisonous plants. However, since the dog scratches himself, the hives soon spread over his whole body.

If this happens to your pet, it is useless to put him on a diet, which won't accomplish anything. Do give him an antihistamine in one form or another: ointment, pill, or injection. People usually have some Phenergan (promethazine hydrochloride) around to ease the discomfort of mosquito bites. Smear the poor bow-wow's entire body with it and, if you have any, also give him some tablets of this powerful sedative. And if need be, give him an injection, as directed (see *Injections,* page 91).

Instead of an antihistamine, you can mitigate the itching by bathing your dog in *cold* water with vinegar in it: 2 bowls of vinegar per 5 quarts (about 5 liters) of water.

In addition, give him a mild sedative. (See *Sedatives,* page 39.)

VACCINES

Every vaccination must be given by a vet and accompanied by a certificate. A puppy represented as having been vaccinated but sold without a certificate of vaccination has not been vaccinated.

(In the U.S., vaccination policies are decided locally, so the pet owner must contact his vet for advice. Most communities require that puppies be vaccinated against distemper and rabies, and kittens against rabies. Vaccines against hepatitis and leptospirosis are also commonly employed. Schedules for vaccinations and boosters vary with the brand name of the drug.—*Trans.*)

WORMS

Ascaris

This small, round worm resembles vermicelli and it usually infests puppies.

This is the easiest disease in the world to detect; as I have already said, the baby dog:

(1) smells as strongly of garlic as if he had eaten a whole clove. (See *Bad Breath,* page 75.)

(2) has a swollen belly, even before eating;

(3) vomits worms which resemble watch springs;

(4) coughs at night (caused by the worms ascending into the throat).

This isn't a very serious condition and there is no reason to worry, but all the same it should be corrected as quickly as possible.

The best way to do so is to go to a druggist and buy a vermifuge for a nurseling, with a piperazine base.

Administer it three days in a row, following the dosage indicated for human babies. In this situation there is no difference between canine babies and human babies.

Add to this vermifuge a mild purgative with a castor oil base. (See *Stopping Lactation* for the proper dose, page 71.)

NOTE: Repeat this treatment every two weeks for at least two months. In licking himself, the puppy gets reinfected and a vicious circle is established unless the disease is eliminated once and for all.

Tenia

There are several types of *Taenia,* the most common being, as in man, the tapeworm—the "solitary worm."

There is another, smaller species which is not solitary at all and which dogs most frequently catch through an intermediate host: the flea.

The dog gets fleas and scratches himself, and when he catches and eats them, at the same time he swallows the microscopic egg containing this miniscule parasite. Much more comfortable in the dog's intestine than in the flea's stomach, the worm develops and grows. This is *Dipilidium caninum.* It has three small flat segments and one large one and is about the size of a melon seed. It's not very dangerous and it is easy to get rid of; you treat it the same way as the tapeworm.

Tapeworm

The tapeworm lives virtually by itself in its home, the intestine. Actually, there is scarcely room for anything else, for it often measures a yard (about a meter).

Dogs in the country have it more often than city dogs. Why? Because rural dogs are often given rabbit intestines or a sheep head, both of which can contain it.

Avoid these two things if you don't want your dog to have a tapeworm.

If he does have one, how do you discover it? Well, usually following an intestinal ailment, you see macaroni-like forms in the dog's stools. These are segments of the tapeworm. The cast-off segments positively do not interfere with the worm's continued existence. Only when the head of the tapeworm has been killed can you be sure that the dog is rid of it.

Garlic, renowned as an old wives' remedy for getting the last of a ribbon of tapeworm, accomplishes nothing.

But pumpkin seeds can be effective. Give the equivalent of a good-sized glass to your pet (see *How to administer a drug,* page 8). They may work; if not you will have to call a vet, who alone will be able to get the last of the huge worm.

In the meantime, your dog may be seized by violent intestinal distress. To relieve this symptom, prepare the following mixture:

7 ounces (about 200 grams, or about 2 glasses) of cold syrup (sugar dissolved in water to the consistency of syrup);

¾ ounce (about 2 tablespoons) of any alcohol you have handy (brandy or 90-proof alcohol);

⅜ ounce (2 teaspoons) of ether.

Give this to your dog (see *How to administer a drug,* page 7). It will settle him down at once—but he will be a little plowed! Allow him to sleep off his liquor in peace.

I knew one dog, a magnificent boxer, who, treated in this manner, developed a taste for this remedy. Like his master, an old paratrooper, the dog was an inveterate alcoholic himself, and the two of them got soused together. Now the dog, when he was drunk, had only one thought in mind: to scratch the inside of his left ear with his right paw, and his right ear with his left paw. Obviously he never succeeded and his efforts resulted in ludicrous antics.

If your dog is drunk after taking his medicine, don't worry about it at all. But even if his discombobulated alcoholic movements make you laugh, don't give him any more just to amuse yourself. A dog who is drunk is as lamentable as a human alcoholic.

NOTE: The syrup prescribed above will settle intestinal upsets but will not kill the tapeworm in the process. It is only a palliative agent to relieve the dog's suffering.

VOMITING

This is a quite frequent occurrence and nothing to be frightened about. Certain breeds with particularly sensitive livers often vomit gastric juice in the morning when their stomachs are empty. (See *Liver Trouble* (*False*), page 52.)

A type of vomiting typical of dogs does exist. The animal eats voraciously; immediately he throws up his meal and eats it again. This isn't very appetizing, I know; however, he should be left alone since this is a normal gastric phenomenon. The dog, having eaten too quickly, hasn't salivated sufficiently for thorough digestion and so the process must be repeated. The dog must throw up what he has just swallowed, in order to eat it again.

Bear in mind that the wolf weans her young in a similar manner. She goes hunting and then carries her booty in her stomach. Returning to her young, she regurgitates the food in front of them, and they eat this meal that their mama has prepared so well for them!

So vomiting an alimentary bolus is normal if it is almost instantaneous.

But there is another kind: when the animal vomits his meal several hours after eating it. This almost always signifies disease: serious liver attack, uremia, metritis, etc.

A vet must be consulted. In the meantime, to counteract the vomiting, if you happen to have a carbonated beverage around, give your pet some. It's miraculous!

Otherwise, give him a good dose of lime blossom tea.

If the vomiting is really intractable and spasmodic, have your dog drink this preparation, which isn't hard to make:

5 grams of ether (1 teaspoon)
5 grams of brandy
110 grams of lime blossom tea (½ cup)
40 grams of orange blossom water (4 tablespoons)
40 grams of chilled sugar syrup: dissolve sugar in cold water until a syrupy consistency is reached.

Mix well and administer 1 teaspoon (small dogs) or 1 tablespoon (large dogs) every 20 minutes. Alternate with a spoonful of mineral water, until the vomiting stops.

INDUCED VOMITING

Sometimes it is absolutely essential to make a dog vomit; for example, if he is poisoned. This is extremely difficult to accomplish.

Of course, you can always try ipecac syrup in these dosages:

1 tablespoon for large dogs,
1 teaspoon for small dogs.

Give this every 10 minutes until the animal vomits. But he won't always do so!

If you don't have any ipecac syrup but you do have some leeks, these may also work, with a little luck.

Huntsmen used to employ this old recipe:

Take the green parts (only) of a bunch of leeks.

Add 1 pint (½ liter) of water and 4 ounces (100 grams) of melted butter to this "brew."

Beat the whole thing until homogeneous and give it to your dog. The dosage will vary according to your patience; give as much as possible, until vomiting ensues. You can also try to get the animal to eat leaves, which have the same property as couch grass, the plant that dogs are so fond of and that makes them vomit.

As with ipecac syrup, this suggestion comes without guarantees. But no matter what happens, *don't* give the dog that famous panacea of our provinces, the handful of salt, which is reputed to induce vomiting. Salt will never induce vomiting, but it may very well aggravate the animal's condition.

‣CATS

HOW TO CHOOSE A CAT

Actually, if you only want a good stray tomcat, you seldom have to buy one. There is always a friend, or a friend of a friend, whose cat has just had kittens that the owner is only too happy to get rid of. Contrary to the case with dogs, there are no "dimwits" among cats to worry about.

Kittens seldom get sick. (See *Constipation in kittens*, page 137.) Just have your kitten vaccinated and then entrust him to Bast, goddess of cats, who will take care of him.

However, if you do have to choose from among several litters, I would advise you that:

White cats, with blue eyes, are always deaf. If they have one blue eye and one of another color (which often happens), they are deaf in one ear only.

Tricolored cats are almost always females. Very occasionally, one will be male, but he will be sterile—although not impotent.

Unicolored cats are very excitable.

Marbled cats are intelligent.

And finally, ginger cats are thieves.

So in theory, the only cats that are purchased—and at very high prices—are the rarer breeds: Siamese, Persians, Abyssinians, Burmese, etc.

These breeds aspire to be the aristocracy of the feline race, and they are all as robust, in the main, as their European relatives. However, contrary to puppies, rarely does one buy them from a retailer. They are usually obtained from a breeder. You may also be able to attend a cat show and make your selection on the spot. There is but one precaution to take, the same as for European breeds: vaccination.

Feeding a cat

A natural hunter and even more of a flesh eater than the dog, the cat is the prototypical carnivore. Vegetables appear to him to be inedible and he looks at your with an air of astonishment when you offer him some. Combat this phobia, beginning when he is quite young. He has less of a need for green vegetables than has the dog, but he has some need for them. When a wild cat eats a bird, he leaves nothing, neither feathers nor viscera; and the latter are filled with vegetable matter in the process of being digested. In this manner the cat takes in the plant matter that he needs, and so you have to provide it to him in another form when he is domesticated. The easiest form in which he will accept this is leeks. But almost all cats are absolutely crazy about asparagus, green beans, and . . . green olives!

Wean a kitten as you do a puppy, by replacing the milk, little by little, with chopped meat mixed with some baby food. This has the advantage of accustoming him at once to the taste of vegetables.

Kittens grow even more rapidly than puppies. At seven months they are adults. So it is necessary to feed them in accordance with their rapid growth:

2 months: 1.8 ounces (about 50 grams) of meat per day, 1.8 ounces of vegetables, an egg yolk every two days, and .35 ounce (about 10 grams) of fat daily; 5 meals per day.

3 to 4 months: 2.7 ounces (about 75 grams) of meat and 2.7 ounces of vegetables daily, an egg yolk every two days, and .7 ounce (about 20 grams) of fat daily; 4 meals per day.

5 to 7 months: 3.6 ounces (about 100 grams) of meat and 2.9 ounces (about 80 grams) of vegetables daily, an egg yolk every two days, and .7 ounce (about 20 grams) of fat daily; 3 meals per day.

Adult: about 7 to 9 ounces (200 to 250 grams) of food per day in two meals.

In order to have a balanced diet, the cat needs more variety than the dog.

Good for him: Lean fish, beef, lamb, liver, poultry, brains, green vegetables. Raw egg yolks are excellent for kittens, pregnant females, and stud males.

To be avoided: milk, when the cat is adult, which will often cause diarrhea; fatty fish (sardines, mackerel); veal; pork.

To be forbidden: Lungs—these familiar "lungs for the cat"— which have no food value; starches; potatoes; spinach greens.

As with dogs, once in a while you can give cats a large beef bone with some meat on which they will enjoy gnawing.

Finally, you can offer them their favorite: catnip (all florists have it but you can make some yourself by dropping a few grains of barley or wheat in a jar). For some unknown reason, they can't leave the stuff alone. If you don't give your cat some, you may catch him eating your flowers or house plants.

Unlike the dog, the cat drinks very little, but he needs very fresh, clear water; even if he hasn't drunk any, change his water two times a day.

Lastly, for cats also there exist prepared foods; but cats are less likely to accept them than are dogs.

HOW TO CARE FOR A CAT

It is harder to handle a cat than a dog. Very supple and lively, this contortionist can turn around, spit out his fury at you, and scratch you before you have time to act.

So employ the element of surprise. Place him on a table and shine a bright light on him as I shall describe below (see *Abscess*, page 122). Then act rapidly before he recovers his orientation. And pet him frequently, especially when handling him. He is very sensitive to petting and tends to forget that anything else is being done to him.

Taking a cat's temperature

See *Temperature*, page 158.

Giving an enema

Inject the liquid and hold the cat's tail between his back paws for several minutes so that the solution isn't expelled immediately.

Giving a suppository

As above, and for the same reason, hold his tail between his paws for several minutes.

Giving liquid

Proceed just as you would for a dog (see *How to administer a drug*, page 8). It is convenient to use a small eyedropper that you insert between his lips. A resistant cat may bite on the eyedropper; if ,so, push it in gently and swallowing will ensue by itself: the act of gnawing forces the animal to swallow.

Giving a pill

Sly cats pretend to swallow their medicine but hide it in their muzzle and spit it out when your back is turned. There is a very simple way to avoid this trick:
First cut up the pill into two or four parts, depending on its size.
Hold the cat's muzzle up and open it. You will then see that his tongue forms a V. Place the pill in the middle of this V. The cat is forced to swallow, reflexly.

Giving a powder

More delicate and discriminating than a dog, if Tabby tastes something questionable in his food, he will reject it. So you can't administer a medicinal powder in this way. Rather, mix it with a sardine drenched in oil. Cats are crazy about sardines in oil and the strong odor of the fish will mask that of the medicine.

Giving an injection

See *Injections,* page 155.

ABSCESS

Certain ailments are more common in some animals than in others, even though they are treated in the same way. This is true of abscesses in cats. Why abscesses particularly? Well, there are two distinctly feline reasons: their needle-like teeth and their claws. When two cats fight, first their claws are unsheathed: each tries to blind the other. Rarely is an eye pierced or even scratched, but abscesses occur rather frequently.

Finally, at the height of the hostilities, each wants to castrate his enemy! This never happens. But the bites are concentrated near the tail, and their teeth are so thin that the holes in the elastic tissue in this region are invisible. The infection festering there assumes the form of an abscess several days later.

I had one customer, a blue Persian of distinguished ancestry, who came to me after every fight, storming and fuming like a curmudgeon: he couldn't abide being put in a basket, even to go to see a vet.

It should be mentioned that he knew himself to be of royal blood, being the son of "Karoun," the famous cat who had served as the model for the mask of the "Beast" in Jean Cocteau's *Beauty and the Beast* and who bore, with much *hauteur,* the title of "King of Cats."

To return to my customer, this worldly cat liked nothing better than to lurk on a rooftop so that he could leap upon those whom he couldn't abide: common cats. Despite their courage, the gutterspout Caesars were beaten, humiliated, and disgraced and having lost face, ran away with their tails lowered in order to hide the wounds to their pride—whereas my customer stuck out his chest, bellowed some disdainful meows, and returned triumphant to his home. But his triumphs came to an end, sooner or later, at my office!

Another of my regulars was a blue and cream Persian who,

despite her marvellous orange eyes, was still a virgin at nine years—which is quite unusual for a cat that hasn't been spayed.

It is true that she was extremely religious, having been raised by a very pious old woman who guarded her cat's virtue vigilantly. Purring their "aves," they said their prayers together every evening.

She had been named, in complete modesty and without any snobbery, "Boudroulboudour," in memory of two lines by the poet J. P. Toulet:

"Have you seen in her palace of adventurine
"Boudroulboudour the Princess of China?"

But outside her adventurine palace, Boudroulboudour liked to climb high up in trees. She pretended to be asleep in order to appease her watchful mistress, and when the latter was reassured and went indoors, Boudroulboudour, her orange eyes reduced to slits, lay in wait for dogs going about their business below.

Choosing the biggest dog who came along, she would jump down on his back. Painfully surprised, he ran away howling. But how could he rid himself of a monster firmly anchored by twenty iron claws to a place that he wouldn't reach? He would turn around but could succeed only in imitating a merry-go-round. When he took off at full speed to escape his torturer he escaped nothing, only carrying his violent pain along with him.

She would "ride" him for two or three miles in this fashion and then, judging that he had been taught a good lesson, she would dismount and return home very satisfied with herself.

Soon all the dogs in the village feared her and no longer came near Mrs. Z.'s house.

For want of canine targets, she threw herself on cats. But this always resulted in a melee and scuffle. Thus it was that the mistress tearfully brought the cat to me: "A horrible alleycat dared attack my poor little pet!"

The Persian, a luxurious animal apparently designed to enter beauty contests, is actually the most ferocious of cats. Other cats are right to do all they can to avoid facing him, but they rarely succeed because he chases them down and makes them fight him. His superior muscularity and the thickness of his fur assure him of having the upper hand and being effectively protected.

The history of these cats, which seems to be authentic, would account for this appetite for fighting.

Around 1800, the docks of Liverpool, where rugs from the Orient were stored, were invaded by rats.

When the importers came to take delivery of their merchandise, only shreds remained: the rats had chewed up the rugs out of hunger.

To fight them, their hereditary enemies were recruited: cats. But the cats succumbed to the multitudes of rats, who attacked by the hundreds. And the dogs that were then thrown into the battle were defeated in the same way. Even men were attacked by these beasts who seemed to have come straight from hell.

This turned into a drama of national proportions. Millions of pounds sterling in the form of rugs were in danger of being gnawed to pieces.

At this point the merchants, faced with ruin, set up a contest for the development of a cat specially bred to hunt rats and to be able to repel them. The requirements were: Fur thick enough to afford protection against bites. Miniscule nose and ears, so that rats wouldn't be able to hang on to them—as they were in the habit of doing. Lastly, strength and ferocity as great as those of their enemies.

Thus it was, apparently, that the Persian resulted from cross-breeding; he was named after the rugs that he saved.

In any event, all cats, including Persians, Europeans, Abyssinians, and Siamese, love to fight, which gives rise to the saying that all cats have abscesses. And all the abscesses are treated in the same manner.

Actually they are treated only when, being sufficiently mature, they open by themselves or can be incised. To bring an abscess to this mature stage apply compresses of very hot and salty boiled water when you notice the little red and inflamed bump which heralds an abscess. The animal will let you do this without protesting. He has no misgivings on this point: he is in pain and quickly understands that hot compresses relieve the suffering.

You can also use a decoction of marshmallow root (boil several pieces of marshmallow for twelve minutes in a little water); this is an excellent emollient that accelerates maturation.

When the abscess is ripe, the center of the bump becomes soft. It is best to take the animal to a vet, who will care for it and make an incision if necessary.

If, for any reason, this is impossible, here is how to proceed:

(1) When you see that the cat is going to develop an abscess, clip the hair over and around the bump.

(2) If by chance the abscess opens by itself, apply hot compresses soaked in boiled water to which you have added several drops of a disinfectant: permanganate or Javel water. The water must be absolutely clear and clean.

If you have to incise the abscess, this won't be easy because the animal may struggle. So it will be to your advantage to find someone to hold the animal.

If you are alone, wrap the cat—including his paws—in a thick towel fastened with safety pins in order to keep him from squirming.

But there is a better way: first put him in a dark place and then, when you are ready to treat him, take him with you into the sunlight or put him under a bright lamp.

A cat's eyes take several minutes to adjust to this sudden change of light. During this interval he can hardly see and he behaves as though hypnotized and doesn't struggle.

If you have to incise the abscess:

(a) Pass a razor blade through alcohol, or through a flame.
(b) With the razor blade, make an incision to the center of the abscess. Pus will escape. Then proceed as described above.

(3) If you have some antiseptic ointment or powder, apply it to the wound. If not, wash it with boiled water into which you have put some Javel water (one teaspoon in a bowl of water) or some hydrogen peroxide. This is perfectly adequate. Abscess wounds which attract white blood cells heal much better than other types. (See also *Wounds,* page 95.)

Tubercular abscess

Man can transmit this disease to cats, and so they often get it. The abscesses are quite characteristic: they can break out anywhere on the body and when they are opened you notice that the pus (which is creamy in normal abscesses) is clotted. Then a kind of ulcer forms on this site which has a tendency not to heal.

NOTE: You cannot do anything yourself but you must consult a vet as quickly as possible.

CAR ACCIDENTS

If a cat is run over by a car, he is usually crushed because of his small size. But there is a chance—a small one—that he will merely be struck and will escape with a broken leg. In such a case he should be cared for like a dog. (See *Auto Accidents*, page 13.)

DELIVERING KITTENS

Cat deliveries are generally uncomplicated. Everything transpires perfectly, only almost always out of human view. Everyone has his modesty—especially a young mother! And everyone also likes to surprise people: to disappear for three days fooling the whole household, and then to return gently carrying in one's muzzle a wet little thing . . . followed by a second . . . then by a third . . . and even a fourth! Fortunately felines rarely have more than four kittens, except for Siamese which are awfully prolific: one of my patients had twenty of them, all dead of course.

An owner's bed also makes a fine lair—and another good surprise!

On the other hand, I once knew a cat who gave birth on the marble of a Louis Philippe secretary, at a convenient height so that the whole family could assemble to witness this entrancing miracle: the birth of a kitten. She purred without interruption through the entire delivery and as each kitten was born she looked at us triumphantly, as if to say, "Did I do that?" One time, because of a clumsy movement and the narrowness of the marble top, she caused one of them to fall to the floor. However, she didn't get alarmed, knowing that the kitten would be picked up; she was, in fact, much less disturbed by the mishap than the people were.

This cat lived with two German shepherds and coexisted cordially with them.

The day following this elevated delivery, the young mother returned to her basket with her newborn kittens. Being traditionalists, the two dogs came to make a churching visit.

The human servant who called herself "mistress" trembled, expecting the cat to be a Fury, her claws way extended. Not at all; around the cradle-basket there was an exchange of girlish and sincere pleasantries. The two female dogs wagged their tails briskly in admiration and sighed sweetly at the little ones. The mother purred proudly, spreading her paws to show them nursing.

Several hours later, the slave-mistress noticed one of the dogs walk past her so cautiously that it seemed strange. Looking more closely, she saw that the animal, its mouth half open, was hiding something black between its lips. Her tender heart skipped a beat—kidnapping? Nothing was in the basket but emptiness: neither cat nor kittens.

The cat hadn't gone far: she was eating contentedly.

Licking her lips heartily, she returned to her basket. How could the bad news be broken to her? She installed herself comfortably, showing no uneasiness at the absence of her little ones. One of the dogs pointed, her tail like a balancing pole and her huge muzzle poised above the cat's delicate abdomen. A purr of gratitude: one kitten had been returned to the fold.

The second dog arrived: the same story. The two babies nursed avidly.

In the days that followed, the facts were simply these: every time the cat went to eat or felt the need to stretch her legs, she consigned her kittens to the dogs, who took them for walks!

It is so unusual for a cat to have trouble with her delivery that you can assume that she should be cared for as you would a dog. (See *Delivering Pups,* page 15.)

NOTE: Occasionally a primiparous cat eats her kittens. This almost always happens in the same way: as the cat cleans the kitten. This is what leads some vets to believe that it is the taste of blood on the umbilical cord that excites the cat and leads her into cannibalism. This behavior also may be due to the abnormal conditions of captivity, particularly with regard to the large felines: lions and tigers in cages often kill their young. Meteorological conditions also seem to play a role: cannibalism in wild animals occurs most frequently toward broods born in winter.

UNDESIRABLE MATING

This is treated as in the dog. (See *Undesirable Mating,* page 24.) But this is difficult to observe: cats are very modest and the sexual act is extremely brief (contrary to the case with dogs).

NURSING

It is rare for a cat not to have milk. If it happens, the kittens must be fed like puppies: the same kind of milk and the same number of feedings. (See *Bottle feeding,* page 28.)

ANEMIA

Anemia is most common in the cat following an internal or external hemorrhage.

This can be detected from two signs, loss of appetite and discoloration of mucous tissues: tongue, lips, gums are of a pale rose—almost white—color. If you cannot reach a vet right away, you should

(1) Sterilize a 10 cc. syringe.

(2) Fill it with physiological saline. (See *Malnutrition,* page 139.)

(3) Inject this solution into the cat four times a day.

If the cat resumes eating, give him a special meaty dish: calves liver or raw chopped beef.

If he refuses to eat, force down some meat juice. To do so, use either a small eyedropper or a plastic syringe. Stick it into the corner of his mouth and inject the fluid slowly. The cat will chew on this unwonted object, and this will induce him to swallow.

NOTE: Anemia in a cat may be due to leukemia, so be sure to consult a vet.

LOCAL ANESTHESIA

Bobeche belonged to some friends. They had adopted her because "Tomcat" was starving himself to death: his beloved mate was no more. In order to save his life they offered him something black and charming and the size of a hedgehog. When she saw him approaching her with shoulders back proudly, she was at once enamored of him.

By and by he came to love his new brown mate very much . . . her abdomen with its dark date color had the same waviness as a woman's hair. But he punished her with abandon whenever she disobeyed their masters!

One Easter Sunday when all the bunnies were about to lay their eggs and the church bells were about to peal, Bobeche, her heart bursting from a thorough and, in her opinion, undeserved licking, decided to mount the wall and go elsewhere to see if all tomcats were so harsh.

Alas, the god of cats punished her for her wicked thoughts. Jumping over the gate, she tore her abdomen badly.

It was her mate who discovered her bleeding, moaning, and promising to be good if only she would be spared. Frightened, he came to get us (I happened to be there at the time).

I examined the long gash.

"It will have to be sewn up."

Since I was on vacation, I hadn't brought anything with me. But a stout needle and some sterile thread were all that were needed (see *Suturing*, page 97).

"You're going to hurt her," moaned the mistress, even more distressed than Bobeche.

"Not if you bring me some ice from your refrigerator," I told her.

Recalling the heroic era of the Napoleonic wars when this was the only anesthetic known, I anesthetized the little cat with some ice cubes that we had intended to use for our whiskey.

Follow my example. When any animal has to be anesthetized and there is nothing else at hand, apply ice. The ice cubes must be applied for a good fifteen minutes to render the area insensitive to pain.

APHTHAE

A client telephoned me one morning: "My cat hasn't eaten for 48 hours and I detected an aphtha on her tongue. I treated her the way I treat myself, with a pinch of bicarbonate, but this didn't accomplish anything and today she is very sluggish."

"Bring her to me at once."

"Why, Doctor? An aphtha isn't very serious."

"By itself, no. But an aphtha in a cat is one of the symptoms of typhus. Take her temperature. I'm sure that your cat's is above 104°F (40°C)."

Ten minutes later my frightened client was in my office with the little creature that fortunately I was able to save.

Don't forget: If your cat refuses to eat and has a fever, examine his mouth. If there is an ulcer at the end of the tongue, there is no mistaking the diagnosis; it is always typhus. (See *Typhus*, page 158.)

Another form of aphtha exists only in older cats. These are actually caused by uremic toxicity. Now uremia, as you may know, is a disease of the elderly. Apply some methylene blue on the aphthae but this is only a symptom and it is the underlying cause that it is essential to treat: the uremia.

Lastly there is the accidental aphtha. Contrary to the preceding type, it is usually the kitten who is susceptible. They find it very amusing to play with plugged in electric cords. Their claws and teeth succeed in wearing through the protective layer and they get an electric shock. If they are lucky, they only receive a burn on the tongue, resulting in an aphtha. (See *Electrical Burns*, page 38.)

Another form of aphtha, harmless in itself, is due to tartar. Disinfect and treat the small sore as you do the preceding, with methylene blue. Once again, you must treat the cause, in this case the tartar. (See *Tartar*, page 102.)

ASPHYXIA

This is treated exactly as in the dog. (See *Asphyxiation*, page 32.)

ASTHMA

This does not occur in the cat. What is referred to as asthma actually is chronic bronchitis. (See *Bronchitis*, page 35.)

ATHREPSIA (Marasmus)

This is a weird story that almost makes one believe in premonitory dreams.

A client of mine gave his wife a four-week-old kitten for her birthday. It had blue-grey eyes that, remarkably, were the same color as its fur.

The young woman was crazy about this ball of fur that curled up on her lap and in her arms and went to sleep purring happily.

Two or three weeks later they were invited to spend a weekend with some friends. They entrusted their little pet to a friendly neighbor and left.

Saturday they had a great time. The weather was beautiful, spring had made the trees blossom, everything seemed perfect.

Sunday morning the young woman suddenly awoke. In her sleep she had just said out loud: "The little cat is dead."

This declaration made first her husband laugh, and then their friends to whom they related the incident. But the young woman didn't laugh. "I am sure that something has happened to Ursus," she repeated, so insistently that Sunday was ruined.

At four o'clock in the afternoon, complaining about "women and their ideas," my client decided to return home, abandoning his friends who wound up being entertained by Molière.

They arrived in Paris. The woman hurried to her neighbor who was upset and immediately told her:

"Your cat has been sick since this morning."

The kitten which had been so gay and lively the night before was lying in a basket. He didn't even seem to recognize the hand that petted him. His hair was dull like paste. Those eyes that had looked out on life so trustingly no longer were open. His breathing was so weak that it seemed about to be snuffed out from one second to the next.

When I arrived, "the little cat was dead," my client was in tears, and the husband was completely floored.

Isn't this astonishing?

"The animal seemed so healthy even yesterday; how could anyone have suspected that he was sick?" my client agonized, upset all the more from having made fun of his wife all day.

But if the dream had been strange, on the other hand there was nothing mysterious about the death itself, bizarre as its circumstances were. The little creature had succumbed to athrepsia. This is a poorly understood ailment with no identifiable cause. It can be related either to intestinal troubles or to worms which subsist on the food that the animal ingests and that make him literally die from hunger. The intractable diarrhea of this disease doesn't help matters any.

The little cat was dead of starvation.

If my client had known more about cats in other than a prophetic sense, she would have quickly noticed that hers was not at all normal. He slept too much for a baby, he wasn't playful enough, but mainly his mucous membranes were completely discolored (as in anemia). When this first occurred, if she had given him some physiological saline, she would perhaps have saved him.

If you ever recognize these symptoms in a young cat, go immediately to a vet, because a young animal has little resistance and you may lose him in a very short time.

If you can't reach one at once, in the meantime give the kitten saline injections, for above all he needs to be rehydrated. Unlike dogs—and camels—cats get dehydrated very rapidly (see *Anemia*, page 128, and *Malnutrition*, page 139). Then check to see if he has worms. If he does, rid him of them at once because they may be responsible for his sickness. (See *Worms*, page 113.)

BURNS

Out in the country I knew two thin-blooded Siamese who had the very bad habit of climbing into the oven when it was turned off but still hot.

One day dreadful screeching was heard: the new maid, ignorant of the ways of the four-legged residents of the house, had shut the door of the oven, trapping the cats inside, and then had lit the stove.

Terrified and bewildered by this screaming roast, she opened the door again and two phantoms engulfed in smoke ran out, heaping insults on her as they ran past. Fortunately they were more afraid than harmed. They were burned most badly on the pads of their paws.

These burns on the bottoms of the paws often occur, in a less dramatic but just as serious manner, from electric ranges. It is usually a naive young cat who, being distrustful of nothing, sets his paw on a hot burner.

Treat the burn as one suffered by a dog. (See *Burns*, page 36.)

SEDATIVES

Be careful using sedatives on cats; unlike dogs, they don't react well to all of them, particularly those that contain benzene. (Always check to see whether or not benzene is an ingredient.)

The same restrictions for dogs regarding aspirin apply to cats. (See *Sedatives*, page 39.)

On the other hand, the cat reacts very well to all barbiturates and these can be given to him without fear. The dosages are:

Adult: the same as for a child.

Kitten: the same as for a nurseling.

UNWANTED KITTENS

A distraught client came to me with a Burmese cat.

"Doctor, you must abort her: she was covered by an alleycat."

"Please understand that it's out of the question. Unlike dogs, cats cannot be aborted without placing their lives in danger," I replied.

"But she is an international champion and I am a professional breeder—it's a catastrophe!"

"Let's not exaggerate. You will give the kittens to some friends and three months later you will marry her, for reasons of state, to a Burmese prince."

"Doctor, you don't understand: she is lost for breeding purposes! Even if she is inseminated by a cat of her breed, now she will always run the risk of having bastards."

Amazing! This is one of those preconceived ideas steadfastly adhered to even though totally false. A single impregnation never stigmatizes an animal. Nothing is left in the womb to affect subsequent litters. Scientifically and medically, this is impossible.

So if a noble cat ever succumbs—the heart has its weaknesses —to the advances of a plebeian, let her have her kittens in peace. Then, if you don't want to keep them, get rid of them.

But please don't do so in a cruel manner. How well I know that for centuries it has been customary to drown kittens, so that this savage practice hardly bothers anyone, even sensitive souls.

I am reminded of an old woman who adored her cat, but not enough to let her keep her kittens. And when I asked her how she intended to get rid of them, she answered calmly:

"Well, I'll throw them down the old toilet and flush it."

This is what is referred to as being kind to animals.

Of course, all along there have been easy ways of killing kittens without making them suffer.

If you own a cheese cover, place them underneath it, along with a large wad of cotton thoroughly soaked with ether. They will go to sleep before dying, but without any pain.

If you have no such bell jar, a box will do just as well, provided that it is perfectly airtight.

FALLS

I knew a charming little Isle of Man cat—one of those famous tailless cats—which was irresistibly attracted to fire and heights.

As for fire—suffering catfish, when he burned his paw a little, he would first spit at the flame and *then* withdraw his paw. And as for heights, he went even further—to be exact, the space between the fourth floor, where he lived, and the sun!

It was impossible to keep track of him by closing all the windows. At least once a month he succeeded in slipping onto the balcony, where he remained for only a couple of seconds.

When his mistress went to scrape him up, he was always very

lively despite his fall of fifty feet and had only one thought in mind: to do it again!

One day, however, she telephoned me in distress.

"Two days ago he fell again as usual, but since then he has been sluggish and sad."

"He must be suffering from slow internal bleeding. Bring him to me; I'll give you a hemostatic agent for him."

Although it is rare to see a cat so drawn to heights, it isn't unusual to see a cat suffer a fall. Two reasons exist for such an accident: love and hunting. A sure-footed feline loses his head just like a clumsy human when he is seized by passion. If in love, he has no thought of risks. As a hunter, he sees only his prey. His eye becomes a telephoto lens that zeroes in for a close-up, generally of a bird; everything else becomes blurred.

I have seen Parisian cats jump through windows to catch pigeons cooing above them. The unfortunate thing is that the sidewalks in cities are of concrete! So instead of just being slightly groggy, the cat will sometimes have an internal hemorrhage or a fractured paw or palate.

Internal hemorrhage

If a cat falls from a height of one story, even if apparently not injured, it is always best to have him examined by a vet. If you are far from one, just to be safe give the animal a coagulant for four or five days (you should always have one in your veterinary medicine kit).

Follow dosage instructions for a child of two to three years.

Fracture of the paw

This is treated like that of a dog. (See *Fracture of the Paw,* page 61.)

Fracture of the palate

This fracture is typical of falls from windows. It is very spectacular but not very serious. The cat lands on his muzzle and the palate is open at the interior like a cockleshell.

Treat this in a simple manner: pat the wound with a large wad of cotton soaked with hydrogen peroxide and don't do anything else. It will heal in several days.

NOTE: During this period of several days *don't give the cat a thing to eat!* The food will get into the nasal passage and cause a serious infection.

On the other hand, you may give him as much water as he cares to drink.

CONSTIPATION

Don't be concerned—especially if your cat is eating only meat—if he only goes to the toilet every two or three days. This is of no consequence; felines are naturally constipated. In fact, wild cats only go once a week!

This is the normal pattern. But if he delays much longer than usual in going to his litter box, this constitutes genuine constipation that should be treated. It usually has one of the following causes:

(1) A hair ball. A cat that likes to keep clean spends part of his time washing himself. Hairs get caught in his little rasp of a tongue and are swallowed. In long-haired cats especially, they collect in the intestine and form a ball that gets stuck there. You can diagnose this condition easily: not only does the cat not go to the toilet but he also refuses all food.

The simplest thing to do in this case is to make him vomit by giving him some baking soda (one good tablespoon in a glass of water) at the rate of one teaspoon every half hour until he vomits up the hair ball.

(2) A poorly functioning liver, often due to the fact that the cat is badly nourished. This is especially common when the cat gets to be around ten years old. Treat this just as you would in a person, with liquid vitamins (see *Giving liquid,* page 121). By all means institute a diet: less meat and a few more carrots.

If the constipation doesn't subside, give an enema.

Administer this by means of an eyedropper (because of the narrowness of the anus), using one part glycerin or paraffin oil to two parts water, preferably cold. (For directions, see *Giving an Enema,* page 121.)

Constipation in kittens

This is usually caused by osteoporosis (see *Osteoporosis,* page 153), an hereditary disease resembling rickets that usually results when consanguineous matings have debilitated the line. In this case administer enemas, but above all take the kitten to a vet who can treat the underlying cause of the constipation, the osteoporosis.

NOTE: *Never* give a cat a laxative for humans: it may kill him, and in any case will make him very sick.

FOREIGN BODIES

Needles

As is well known, cats adore spools of thread. Unraveling them amuses them much more than their mistresses enjoy sewing, and mixing up the ends of spools of thread seems to be their favorite pastime. This form of entertainment can prove dangerous; for example, when a needle is stuck in the spool of thread.

In such an event, arm yourself with a pair of tweezers, hold the animal's mouth open, and pull out this needle that has mistaken his tongue or palate for a pincushion.

Occasionally a needle becomes lodged vertically between the tongue and palate: the poor little cat is sewn together. In order to unstitch him you have to lift the needle out carefully, making sure not to break the needle in the flesh—which would make the operation much more difficult.

In the throat

See *In the throat* under Dogs, page 43.

In the mouth

See *In the mouth* under Dogs, page 44.

In the ears

See *"Potatoes" in the ears,* page 45.

COMMON COLD

It was three o'clock in the morning when I was awakened by a phone call. A frail voice apologized for having awakened me and said:

"My cat is suffocating, Doctor; he is dying before my very eyes! Would you let us see you right away, despite the late hour?"

The voice sounded so distressed and miserable that I agreed.

Twenty minutes later, my bathrobe over my pajamas, I received a very charming old lady accompanied by a no less charming cat—who didn't seem at all bent on dying.

"I don't understand it at all," said his mistress, all upset. "When I called you, he was at the end of his rope! That's why I allowed myself to . . . ."

It was I and my conscience that were at the end of our rope. However, since the "dying patient" was there, I figured I might as well examine him. He himself was proceeding to examine my living room, which seemed to interest him greatly.

"He has a good cold," I said. "In cats, that's an infectious and quite serious disease. He is having trouble breathing the way you do when you get a head cold. I imagine that your apartment is good and warm?"

"Yes; at my age, Doctor, I like warmth."

"Yes but in that overheated atmosphere, inflamed mucous membranes get even more congested and that is what caused your cat to have trouble breathing. Furthermore, the anxiety associated with having trouble breathing itself aggravates the discomfort. The fresh outdoor air, coupled with the distraction of going somewhere, have given him a temporary respite. But as soon as you return home he'll have trouble again. Only one thing will ease this condition: an inhalant."

She looked at me with great consternation.

"But how . . . he would never agree to that! I wouldn't be able to do it."

Given her age I thought she might have one of these handy old lye washers, which unfortunately have gone out of style.

She did have one but she stared at me with her eyes open wide in astonishment. That a veterinarian should discuss lye washing with her at three o'clock in the morning seemed more than a little strange.

"Well," I told her, "you should prepare a fumigator as you would for yourself, and when it starts to boil, place the fuming liquid in the bottom portion of the lye washer. Cover this bottom part with the kind of perforated lid that you usually place under the fabric, and then put your cat inside the lye washer for a quarter of an hour. The fumes of the inhalant will escape through the holes and he will be forced to inhale it."

So if you have a cat afflicted by a good cold, don't forget that:

(1) He is very miserable because the nose of a cat (especially a Persian) is small and so it gets stuffed up readily.

(2) In cats, coryza is a serious disease that must be treated assiduously from the beginning if you wish to prevent bronchitis or even bronchial pneumonia. If you cannot reach a vet who can give the cat antibiotics, expose the animal to a fumigator. This is the only effective remedy.

If you don't own a lye washer, place a small box pierced with holes inside a larger box, and proceed as above. The bowl containing the liquid is placed inside the small box, the cat inside the large one.

Ready-made inhalants are available at the pharmacy but you can make one up yourself by boiling together one part eucalyptus leaves and one part marshmallow root. Eucalyptus is an excellent disinfectant and marshmallow root is the best of emollients.

As for the cat in the lye washer, don't forget about him and boil him!

MALNUTRITION

The cats in the huge cage at the pound didn't even think about rough-housing. Their eyes peering out through the wire mesh, they all waited patiently and beseechingly for whoever was going to save them. They seemed to know that if no one came for them, certain death awaited them.

Heartbroken, the young woman looked at them. She was going to rescue one of them. She was in despair over the thought that she would be leaving all the others to their fate. They came out of their mental depression and crowded together toward her, meowing and begging, "Me."

It was then that she noticed "him." Perched atop a kind of bench, his long tail hanging down, his golden eyes were barely open as though he didn't want to look at her. Proud of his black Angora heritage, he refused to be associated with this mendicant rabble.

"He's the one I want!"

The good woman who looked after the animals looked askance.

"Since we've had him, he has refused to eat. I think he's going to starve himself to death! I doubt that you'd be able to save him."

"He's the one I want!"

And the young woman carried the Angora away like a stolen treasure, turning her back on all the others she was abandoning.

Arriving home, the black cat purred but refused a saucer of milk: after a week of fasting, he had forgotten that he had to eat. He also declined the meat offered him.

It was Sunday. The only vet in the small town was off duty.

The young woman was a nurse by trade. She pondered the situation: what would be done for a patient in such a case? Physiological saline, or course! All the drugstores were closed, but a nurse knows what physiological saline is made of; it's very simple. So she prepared some and, unable to administer it drop by drop to an animal, she gave him an injection every two hours.

The next day she took him to another nurse, who later told me this story. He could only tell her she had done the right thing and encourage her to continue.

The cat had malnutrition; as the popular phrase puts it so aptly, his stomach was shrunken. Moreover, his lassitude due to the lack of nourishment prevented him from extending the effort necessary to save himself. It was a vicious circle. He had to be fed in order to restore his strength and desire to eat. This was the idea behind the physiological saline.

If a cat has malnutrition, he should be given saline injections and treated for anemia. (See *Anemia,* page 128.)

Physiological saline can be made up by anyone, as long as the *proper concentration* is maintained. If not, it can be fatal.

This concentration is two level teaspoons of salt per liter (1.06 quarts).

Boil this solution for three minutes and then cool before you administer it.

Don't forget that physiological saline is used in all illnesses requiring rehydration.

DEHYDRATION

I have good reason to remember the winter of 1963 and to recall that it was especially frigid. At the end of December of that year, some clients of mine and their cat went for a weekend in the country. When they were about to return—no more cat! His masters called him and looked everywhere, all in vain. After two hours they had to come to the inevitable conclusion: Mickey had disappeared. Had someone kidnapped him in order to make him into a stew? Had he left of his own free will? A mystery. With heavy hearts they returned home.

The following week came the great cold wave: snow, icy roads impairing traffic, and in Paris the thermometer plummeted to 7°F (−14°C)—very low for that area.

Three weeks later the thaw came and my clients returned to their country house to survey the damage that the freeze had caused.

Checking everything, they opened a little tool shed at the foot of the garden. A ghost ran out: Mickey! As flat and dry as a board, the cat was still alive nonetheless. By what miracle? A candle should have been lit for Saint Francis of Assisi.

The animal had lived for three weeks without eating and without drinking, from the time he had been shut inside. This was most remarkable since the cat is an animal that gets dehydrated very rapidly.

An hour later they came to me with Mickey, all dried out.

Immediately I injected some physiological saline into him. At the end of two days, the little cat had "reinflated" and regained his feline contours.

The same experience may happen to you. With tneir mania for getting into closets and hiding there so they can sleep in peace, cats often cause themselves a problem like this.

In such an event, before giving the little thing something to eat or drink, check and see if he is dehydrated: pinch the skin of his neck. If the layers of skin remain together and don't exhibit their usual elasticity, before you do anything else—even before taking him to the vet, because this may be a matter of seconds—give him some 4 cc. injections of physiological saline, repeating them every hour. If you don't have any, you can prepare it yourself. (See *Malnutrition,* page 139.)

Don't forget: This measure may save your pet's life.

POISONING

With shórt and bushy blue-grey fur, innocent blue eyes, a long tail held very erect, and the air of a dandy, this "Russian blue" was going on eight months. The "ideal" age. The gentle, purring kitten, his head lying on his paws, actually was always trying to think up ways of driving his master to distraction!

This particular day he had found a little bottle in the bathroom and, taking advantage of the fact that no one was around, he had struck it with his paw and knocked it over. Many tiny marbles fell out that the cat trapped in the hollow beneath his paw and then brought to his mouth. Accidentally he swallowed one of them.

A half hour later his master returned to find Blue curved in the form of an arc, and rigid. This strange position was followed by an abrupt reversal in the opposite direction, and then the cat loosened up and became almost normal. He placed his paw on his master's hand as if to ask for help; animals do make such gestures. Beside him was the bottle emptied of its little pellets which were of none other than a tonic with a strychnine base.

As you might imagine, Mr. R. was frightened and telephoned me.

"Bring him to me at once! He will survive five seizures, no more. The last will be fatal!"

Then I realized that by the time that he got here the little creature would be dead.

"Have you any phenobarbital?" I asked.

By chance, Mr. R. did have some.

"Give him an injection of it immediately; it will delay the second attack."

But Mr. R. had only pills. So I described the emergency treatment to him:

(1) Boil some water for three minutes. You then have some sterilized water and a sterilized instrument (the saucepan in which you boiled the water).

(2) Simultaneously, boil a syringe and a needle in another saucepan.

(3) Leave about one tablespoon of boiled water in the saucepan and dissolve the phenobarbital in it, liquid or tablet form, (the dosage is the same as that taken by mouth). (See *Sedatives*, page 39, for the proper dosage.)

(4) When the medicine is dissolved, draw the solution up in the syringe and give the injection normally.

Of course, you may get—probably will get—an abscess at the injection site. But what is an abscess compared to death?

Don't forget: If an animal is poisoned with strychnine, the only antidote is phenobarbital.

Obviously, strychnine poisoning is rare. Nevertheless, in rural areas some old-timers still use a powder with a strychnine base against field mice.

On the other hand, dogs and cats are poisoned more and more frequently by herbicides, defoliants, and insecticides. Don't fool yourself, an animal's size doesn't help him resist these chemicals any better than the caterpillars, slugs, or weeds do.

Poisoning with herbicides

See *Poisoning with herbicides* under Dogs, page 58.

Poisoning with arsenicals

Arsenic is contained in many gardening products. You can tell right away if your pet has swallowed some: he smells as strongly of garlic as you do when you have eaten a garlic dressing; there is no mistaking it. So if ever you suspect that he has taken in some arsenic, open his muzzle and smell.

Of course, this sign will be rapidly succeeded by the symptoms of arsenic poisoning: spasms, vomiting, diarrhea.

Immediately give the animal some egg whites beaten in milk; milk is the antidote for arsenic.

And if you happen to have some: limewater (see *Diarrhea in a puppy,* page 75) or, instead, magnesia water.

Lastly, a cardiac stimulant should be given. For cats this is tea and for dogs, coffee.

Poisoning with metaldehyde (antigastropod agents)

This is the sweet death of the slug. No one knows why he loves his poison, but it's a fact that he does. If you wish, you can see this for yourself, as I myself did. As a young camper, I had a portable metaldehyde stove, and every morning I found 30 or 40 dead slugs near it.

Metaldehyde is no better for your cat. If he ingests some, the effects begin to be felt a half hour later: he will be seized by drooling and then by vomiting, spasms, and muscular rigidity. If this should happen to him and you have been spreading an anti-gastropod agent in your garden, have no doubts as to what has happened and act at once. To do so:

(1) Induce vomiting, either with some ipecac (one teaspoon every five minutes until it works) or with baking soda. (See *Constipation,* page 136.)

(2) As soon as he has vomited, give him about ⅓ ounce (10 grams) of sodium sulfate so that the poison can be evacuated as fast as possible (for a dog, about 1¾ ounces, or 50 grams). In carnivores, sodium sulfate has an immediate effect.

(3) Give him an injection of phenobarbital (see *Poisoning,*

page 142) or any other barbiturate instead. (I say injection deliberately: in tablet form he will expel it when vomiting.) This will inhibit his spasms and muscular rigidity.

(4) After he has vomited, give him some medicinal charcoal. If you have none make some by burning some bread until it is completely charred. Carbon has the property of absorbing toxic gases.

Lastly, metaldehyde poisoning almost always has nephritis as a sequela.

NOTE: New products are being used more and more. Gardening products have their formula indicated on the package. So don't throw it away, and take it to the vet if your pet is poisoned. This can make the difference between saving the animal and not.

The vet will telephone a poison control center, which will immediately advise him on the antidote to give. If you can't reach a vet, call such a number yourself in an emergency.

Poisoning with insecticides

DDT is extremely toxic to a cat. It is contained not only in insecticide powders but also frequently in ear drops. Before using either one, always check the formula to be sure that it doesn't contain DDT.

In any case, prevent the animal from licking himself after each powdering of his fur and brush him after a half hour—thoroughly enough that no powder remains in his fur.

If a powder containing DDT is mistakenly used, this will quickly become apparent. The feline will be seized by convulsions, will fall down, and may even go into cardiac arrest. DDT doesn't kill only fleas, it also kills cats, especially if you keep using the same toxic powder.

In such a case give the animal:

(1) A sedative with a barbiturate base. (See *Sedatives*, page 39.)

(2) Some sodium sulfate to bring about elimination of the

poison, in the dose indicated (see *Poisoning with metaldehyde,* page 144).

(3) Injections of physiological saline (see *Malnutrition,* page 139).

(4) A little strong tea (which is an excellent cardiac stimulant for the cat).

NOTE: Above all, don't give him any milk. This, as well as oil, is contraindicated.

Poisoning with acid

As I have already warned, one never knows what a young pet will get into. While playing, a cat or dog may swallow some acid. Various household products contain acids; for example, spirits of salt and—much less dangerous—vinegar.

The symptoms are very clear and there is no mistaking them:

(1) inflammation of the mucous membranes
(2) drooling
(3) vomiting
(4) spasms.

If the condition isn't treated *immediately,* holes will be burned in the stomach and intestine. Death is the result.

Therefore, *before anything else,* give an alkaline substance. This may be, in order of importance:

(1) Egg whites beaten in limewater (see *Diarrhea in a puppy,* page 75).

(2) Hydrated magnesia.

(3) Soapy water (one tablespoon of grated soap per quart—about a liter—of water) in as large a quantity as you can get him to accept (at least ½ pint—¼ liter—for a small animal; 1 pint—½ liter—for a large one).

Give this with either a syringe or an eyedropper.

NOTE: Don't induce vomiting in the animal by giving emetics!

Poisoning with detergents

While playing, a young animal may knock over and swallow some detergent—extremely potent—which is used to scour enamel (toilets, bathtubs, etc.). In this event, the treatment is the same as for acids.

Poisoning with alkali (ammonia, lye, etc.)

The symptoms are identical to those of acid poisoning—vomiting, salivation, etc. In addition, there are signs of asphyxia due to edema around the glottis (i.e. swelling around the throat). As with alkali burns, treat alkali poisoning with a neutralizing chemical, namely an acid: lemon juice or vinegar. Obviously it won't be very easy to get your pet to swallow this, but it can be done (see *Giving liquid,* page 121).

Poisoning with nicotine

A retired man had some rosebushes that were his pride and joy. The rosebushes had aphids. The old man extinguished his cigarette butts in the water which was then sprinkled on the flowers. The aphids were killed by the nicotine, which is a poison. (Doctors are certainly correct in trying to combat the use of tobacco.)

The pensioner, however, also had a cat that he loved and about whom he called me because it had fallen ill.

At the foot of the rosebushes was a nice patch of grass in which Puss regaled herself. However, some of the nicotine vapor fell on the grass and the cat was poisoned just like the aphids.

If something like this should happen to your cat, you should:

(1) Make the cat vomit. (See *Induced Vomiting,* page 117.)
(2) Get him to swallow some medicinal charcoal, either voluntarily or by force. (See *Poisoning with metaldehyde,* page 144.)

(3) Put him on an all-dairy diet until completely cured—milk is the antidote for tobacco.

NOTE: All poisonings *no matter what are very serious* and can be fatal. Therefore, after giving first aid, show the animal to a vet.

EPILEPSY

See *Epilepsy* in Dogs, page 60.

A cat is very rarely truly epileptic, but the use of DDT as an insecticide (see *Poisoning with insecticides,* page 145) often is responsible for a pseudo-epileptic-attack.

This condition may also be due to ear mange. The insufferable itching that this causes literally drives the cat crazy. (See *Itchy ears,* page 84.)

EXTENSION OF THE SPINAL COLUMN

The mistress groaned disconsolately: the beautiful silk that covered the walls of the living room had been scratched away over an entire panel by the little white cat that had been "filing her nails" on it.

"But I always cut them with a nail clippers," she told me, sadly recounting her misfortune. "So she didn't have to do that."

"Yes she did, because 'filing her nails' has two purposes for a cat. The first is obviously to blunt nails that have grown too sharp, but the second is to provide the cat with a gymnastic exercise!"

This latter function is very important for the animal's vertebral column. This is why even if his nails are worn down, he will practice this extension movement.

In order to allow him to do this without ruining your chairs or drapes, provide him with a piece of a tree branch. Some Sunday when you are out in the country, bring one back and nail it upright in a corner of his favorite room—upright to allow him to make this extension movement.

EYE AILMENTS

The cat's vision

An antique dealer, the owner of a gorgeous chinchilla, said to me:

"I'm scared to death. At night he walks on top of my opaline table. I have some irreplaceable pieces; if he should knock over even one of them . . . ! During the day he would be able to see his way around—but he never goes exploring then! He only climbs up when it's dark."

I had to laugh. "Has he broken anything yet?"

"Never. It's really a miracle!"

"Not at all; he can see then almost as clearly as you can during the day. The popular belief that cats can see at night is perfectly true. Unlike the dog, this little feline has exceptional vision."

Furthermore he is guided by his whiskers, which are tactile hairs of exquisite sensitivity.

The third eyelid

On the one hand, there is the third eye hallowed by Tibetan lamas and monks; and then there is the third eyelid, which actually exists in cats. It is also found in dogs, and even in man. But since man is an animal in decline, only a trace of it remains in him.

This is actually the nictitating membrane, which is located at the internal angle of the eye and which separates it from the external eyelid. It is functional in all mammals but especially in felines; that is why I am describing it now, for I shall have to refer to it below.

In order to view this third eyelid, you hold the upper eyelid up and push in gently with your finger; you will then see the nictitating membrane stand out.

Blurred vision in a cat

The storm was about to break out for sure. The weather vane, facing in an ominous direction against a depth of threatening black clouds, confirmed the fact; the heat was intolerable; and in the still grass not even an insect could be heard.

It was as agonizing as the approach of a cataclysm.

Lying with his paws curled under him, Blacky had never looked so much like a fortune teller's cat. Storms terrified him. His mistress leaned over to stroke his soft fur, which crackled from the static electricity in the air.

The little creature didn't purr but raised his violet eyes toward the young woman.

She screamed, "Blacky has gone blind!"

Frightened and mystified, she gazed at him. What had happened to the green highlights that made people say that Blacky had the most beautiful eyes in the world? A veil completely shrouded them.

"Cataracts," thought Mrs. R.; "but in both eyes? And how come I didn't notice them sooner?"

While pondering the situation, she got her cat's basket, shoved him inside unceremoniously and tossed the basket into her car. Then, in the torrential rain that was falling at last and amid the bellicose tom-tom of thunder, she drove to the vet.

There were one or two people in the waiting room. Her voice trembling, she asked:

"This is an emergency; will you let me go first?"

She appeared so upset that the other clients agreed at once.

She set the basket on my desk and before even opening it, she told me:

"Blacky is blind."

"I see," said I, thinking of course of an accident. "What happened to him—a fight with another cat?"

She opened the lid of the basket and the cat darted toward me, an angry green glow in his eyes.

"But . . . it's a miracle!" Mrs. R. exclaimed, absolutely stupefied.

And she told me what had happened.

There had been no miracle. It was spring; Monsieur Cat's eyes had gotten this "blurriness" which was further aggravated by the storm.

By a physical phenomenon familiar to all vets, the third eyelid comes over the eye in this condition.

This is what had happened to Blacky. His anger at being put in his basket, his distraction from being carried about, the end of the storm—all these factors combined to dissipate this blurriness, permitting him to recover his vision at the same time.

If this should happen to your cat, it is futile to take him to a vet or to get worried. This is a natural phenomenon that will go away by itself.

Cataract

Cats, who have excellent vision, rarely have cataracts, but if your cat should, proceed as for a dog. (See *The dog's vision,* page 76.)

Conjunctivitis

See *Conjunctivitis,* page 77.

Eczema of the eye region
See *Dog "wearing glasses,"* page 79.

Thorn in the eye

See *Thorn in the eye,* page 78.

Scratched eye

Two cats fight. A painful swat with a paw and there is a scratch on the eye.

The animal has to be taken to the vet immediately, of course, but first several drops of methylene blue have to be put in the eye also. (See *Scratched eye,* page 79.)

Ulcerated cornea

See *Ulcerated cornea,* page 79.

BAD BREATH

As in the dog, this may be due to digestive causes. (See *Bad Breath,* page 82.) More often, by dental tartar.

In licking himself, a cat pulls out some of his hair. This hair—especially if it is long—gets stuck to the tartar, and from that moment on, a veritable odor of putrefaction emanates from his darling little pink mouth.

In the cat, as in the dog, tartar is a result of an overcivilized existence.

A wild cat that hunts and kills a bird or mouse tears the flesh from it limb by limb in order to eat, and at the same time he cleans his teeth.

But mushy catfood or finely chopped meat requires no effort; the cat swallows it without even having to chew. Particles of this food remain between his teeth, giving rise to tartar and bad breath. To prevent this, rub the cat's teeth with a lemon (see *Tartar,* page 102) and from time to time give him a bone to gnaw.

If you do this regularly, there will never be any tartar deposits.

Certain breeds of cat get this more easily than others: Persians, and cats with red hair. Why redheads? No one knows, but it's a fact!

On the other hand, Siamese cats—if they are pure—almost never get tartar; neither do Europeans. These two breeds have good-looking and healthy teeth.

Persians get their long hair caught between their teeth and almost go crazy trying to get rid of it with their paws. In such a case you have to help them by pulling it out with a pair of tweezers.

If you haven't followed my advice and your pet gets tartar, it must be removed by a vet. (See *Tartar,* page 102; and also *Ascaris,* page 113.)

SNAKEBITE

This is extremely rare, since cats are usually much quicker than snakes.

If by chance this should occur, treat the animal as you would a dog. (See *Snakebite* in Dogs, page 85.)

INGROWN TOENAILS

This happens to very old housecats that don't have the strength to "file their nails." The nails get long and curve around like all feline nails, and they wind up penetrating the footpads. The animal suffers greatly and can no longer walk. So he has to be taken to a vet, who will clip his nails and remove the points embedded in the flesh.

To prevent this very painful condition, cut the nails. A cat usually allows you to do this very readily, especially if you have done this regularly since he was a kitten.

To do so:

(1) Seat the animal on your knees.

(2) Take a paw in your left hand and push lightly on the footpads in order to make the nails spring out.

(3) Then clip the ends with a nail clippers. Never use scissors, which may slip and injure the animal.

(4) Repeat with the other paw.

NOTE: The distal phalanx (last finger bone) is inserted into the cornified sheath that holds the nail. So you only have to blunt the nail; if you cut it too close you'll cut this last phalanx. This can be done intentionally to prevent nail growth completely, but this procedure, which is done on wild cats and housecats, is exclusively the province of the veterinarian.

OSTEOPOROSIS

This Abyssinian knew that she was the true descendant of a goddess. She vaguely remembered that famous age when a devout people came "by land and water," as recounted by Herodotus, to her temple to worship her. Hundreds of thousands held great feasts in her honor: she was Bast, daughter of Ra the sun god and goddess of joy.

From this extraordinary past she had retained the hieratic quality of Egyptian art, and the nobility and indulgence of those who had received these prayers and supplications so long ago.

Like certain large wild beasts, the Abyssinian's fur has three shades: white, brown, and maroon. Together with her panther-like agility, this doubtless is why a ferocity has been attributed to her which is completely alien to her.

A trifle lost in the world of humans, the cat goddess has become somewhat shy of them. When a person lucky enough to have an Abyssinian lodger entertains guests, the cat disappears. She only emerges from her Olympian retreat when her human friend is alone again.

Not long ago, then, her master brought to me the cat that he had named Bast in honor of her Egyptian origin.

"She must have sprained her paw jumping down from a piece of furniture; see how she is limping."

No, unfortunately, my Abyssinian friend had something much more serious than a sprain. She suffered from osteoporosis, which is almost the equivalent for cats of what arthritis is for people, except that it affects the bones and not the joints.

It strikes Abyssinians and Siamese particularly; that's why the latter breed so often has a bumpy tail. Contrary to popular belief, a twisted tail in a Siamese isn't proof at all that he is purebred, only that he suffers from osteoporosis.

This is a painful and incurable disease. Only a vet can treat an animal that is affected and minimize the damage.

I mention this here even though this is never a matter of emergency, because the owner of the animal often diagnoses it incorrectly. Seeing his pet limp, he thinks he only has rheumatism; but osteoporosis is a disease of kittens and kittens seldom get rheumatism.

If you have an Abyssinian or a Siamese, bear in mind that more than most cats he is subject to osteoporosis. Take him to the vet at the first symptoms, before it is too late. This serious disease, if not treated in time, can cause total paralysis of the animal.

LACK OF OXYGEN

To administer oxygen to a cat, it is best to enclose him in a large box in which a hole has been made for the tank hose. (See also *Lack of Oxygen* in Dogs, page 87.)

DRESSING OF WOUNDS

See *Dressing of Wounds* for Dogs, page 88.

INJECTIONS

Proceed exactly as with a dog (see *Injections*, page 91), the cat's back being comparable to that of the rabbit in being readily accessible for an intramuscular injection.

Subcutaneous injections can be safely made in the thick skin of the neck where the cat's mama used to grip him when carrying him. This not only is the best place to make a subcutaneous injection, it is also the best place to hold him because, even if you are without assistance, he won't turn around: he is "tranquilized" as he was when his mother carried him in this manner. Moreover, regressing to an infantile state because of this tactile stimulation, he takes on a sense of inferiority and doesn't dare to rebel. (In many mammals, stimulation of the neck region causes passivity, mediating "playing possum" to deceive predators as well as facilitating transport by the mother. This sensitivity may also be exploited by males to pacify females in coitus, even in our own species.—*Trans.*)

FUR

The little cat had "queasiness." He was fussy just like infants that have indigestion and refuse all food.

Because he was very clean and liked to look his best, the long-haired Persian made his toilet every morning.

His rough pink tongue glided through his fur, combing it out and meticulously removing the dead hair—which he swallowed! The result: a ball of hair totally blocked his intestine.

This can be quite serious because if it isn't removed it will lead to intestinal obstruction. So vomiting must be induced.

There is a very simple and effective means of doing this, used by all breeders: baking soda.

In a glass of water, dissolve as much sodium bicarbonate as possible: it takes about two good tablespoons to reach the saturation point.

Then administer the sodium bicarbonate to the cat on a schedule of one teaspoon every ten minutes until he vomits.

This may happen very quickly, or it may take a very long time. Be patient and keep going until the hair ball (which usually takes the shape of the stomach) is rejected.

If this doesn't work—always a possibility—you will have to extricate the hair through the "rear exit." This is where paraffin oil comes in. As a last resort, the vet will prescribe some eserine salicylate or a similar drug for you.

RICKETS

The darling little Siamese cat was named Dove. Wishing to be true to her name, she retracted her claws in order to cuddle up to her owners. But she couldn't stop herself from sticking them out when she saw something unusual that displeased her. The Siamese is a true wild animal and reacts like one. He looks as if he were descended from a leopard whose dark spots slipped to the tips of his tail, paws, and ears.

Dove was married, very properly, to a Siamese tomcat who lived under the same roof, and she regularly presented him with six kittens . . . six times a year.

Although the European cat is content to have four litters of four kittens each (which in itself is not bad), the Siamese and the Abyssinian—great earth mothers both—are only satisfied with three dozen annually.

Recently her mistress brought the last litter to me. She was terribly disappointed: the kittens had Louis XV paws, backbones like roller coasters, and knotted tails (contrary to common belief, the Siamese should have a straight tail).

"They all have rickets," she told me.

She was wrong about that. Cats never have rickets but they do get osteoporosis (see *Osteoporosis*, page 153), which is mistaken for rickets.

"Dove had too many babies," I told her. Osteoporosis comes from being worn out; unfortunately it is a disease that attacks the offspring of overly fecund felines.

In such a case there is only one remedy, a radical one. The cat must be spayed so she has no more kittens (see below) and, alas, the affected litter should be put to sleep.

RABIES

See *Rabies* in Dogs, page 99.

STERILIZATION

Hardly a day passes without my door opening to reveal a little sweetheart:

"Doctor, I've brought her to you to be 'fixed.'"

Unlike human "sweethearts," the cat cannot take the pill. So there is only one solution for such an unrepentant sinner: sterilization.

Obviously, this safe procedure should only be performed by a vet. I mention it here because I have noticed that my clients have some totally erroneous ideas about it.

Thus, most believe that the animal should have had at least one litter before being "fixed," which is absolutely false.

There are actually two ways to proceed:

The French method: the operation is performed after the cat has gone into heat for the first time (at about six months).

The American method: you operate before the first estrus.

It goes without saying that you can perform this procedure on a cat which has given birth once or several times.

Temperature

Unless he is very gentle and is used to having you take care of him, it is always quite difficult to take the temperature of a cat, an animal cautious by nature.

Wait until he is lying down or asleep—preferably both—before trying to do so. Petting him throughout, lift up his tail and, after having taken the precaution of smearing the area with vaseline, introduce the end of the thermometer into the anus. Beware of a reflex reaction from his claws or teeth, however!

Unlike the dog's, the cat's temperature is stable. Normally it is 100.4°F (38°C). Anything above this constitutes a fever, but anything below this is ominous also, since it may indicate poisoning.

TOXOPLASMOSIS

See *Toxoplasmosis* in Dogs, page 104.

NOTE: It is probable that cats, like dogs, transmit toxoplasmosis to man.

TUMORS

See *Tumors* in Dogs, page 108.

TYPHUS (Leucopenia)

Several years ago in a German zoo, a panther befriended a stray cat that had come, fearlessly, to pay her a visit. And why not? The one had a very large handsome body, the other a very small one, but they were still both felines who purred together in unison! They had the same coat of black silk, the same topaz eyes. Perhaps the panther believed that she was realizing the dream of every mother: to have a little one that never grows up.

At first the cat, rather unsociably, hid when the keeper brought the big beast her food. But the tempting smell of meat won him over. He meowed that he would very much like to be invited to lunch; all the same, he wasn't going to invite himself to dine amidst the powerful claws of his companion. The firmest friendship can be turned sour by such a *faux pas*.

The keeper, a kind soul, faithfully brought two servings at noon: a quarter of beef for the wild animal, and a bit of lungs for the cat.

When night fell the little feline slipped between the bars and went to search for excitement on the rooftops. At dawn he re-entered the cage where the forlorn beast snarled in frustration at not having been able to accompany him. But one morning he returned with such slow, labored steps that the panther realized that he had had to summon all of his loyalty to return to her side.

When the keeper came at noon carrying the two lunches, she was crazed with grief and didn't even let him approach the cage where the thin body of the cat was lying.

For three days the beast refused all food. Downcast and despairing, she lay curled up in a corner, not even opening her eyes.

On the fourth day, she went to Animal Heaven to rejoin her friend. . . .

The keeper was convinced that she had let herself die from grief.

The vet was somewhat less certain, and he proved to be right. The cat, an incorrigible tramp, had caught typhus, the most contagious of all feline diseases. His friendship for the wild beast, in turn, had killed her: by returning to die near her, he had transmitted the disease to her.

This story of stray cats having typhus and transmitting it to the wild animals is now so well known that in every zoo the big cats are vaccinated against this terrible disease.

If you have a cat, take the same precaution, particularly if you live in the country where the animal can run freely. (See *Vaccines*, page 113.)

Typhus in a cat is entirely different from the disease in dogs (who cannot infect one another), but it is just as deadly because it causes complete destruction of white blood cells. When this happens, the animal has no more resistance.

If he hasn't been vaccinated, you will be able to tell that he is sick by the following symptoms:

(1) Lethargy and prostration.
(2) A very high fever that goes up to 105.8°F (41°C) and lasts for three days.

You thus have 48 hours in which to get the stricken animal to a vet. Any later than that will be *too* late.

MEDICINE CABINET (for a Dog and a Cat)

90- or 60-proof alcohol
An antibiotic—the already old reliable penicillin-streptomycin combination (one million units and one gram) is recommended; for the cat, tetracycline in tablet form
    aspirin
    elastic and nonelastic bandages
    a barbiturate
    methylene blue in solution
    a sedative—potassium bromide solution, for example
    medicinal charcoal
    scissors—preferably with blunt ends
    gauze compresses—preferably sterile
    cotton
    hydrogen peroxide—replenish frequently
    ether—replenish because it evaporates
    ipecac—in medicinal syrup form
    tweezers
    Phenergan (promethazine hydrochloride)—a vial of tablets
    a diuretic—with a base of lactose, strophanthus, etc.
    a hemostatic and "coagulant: for external use"
    a sulfonamide powder
    bismuth salts for the intestine; for example:

        bismuth subnitrate, tannoform, and benzonaphthol—⅙ gram each or:
        bismuth subnitrate and prepared chalk (½ gram each) plus opium powder (50 milligrams)

10-milliliter syringe and ⁸⁄₁₀-section needle—the shortest possible size so that the injection can be made even if the animal struggles

antisnakebite serum—prepared by local agencies to suit the snakes of the region

tincture of iodine—fairly fresh: it changes with time

thermometer

cardiotonic agent (camphorated oil)

trocar

small eyedropper

These items are not all sold without a prescription, so you'll need to ask a practicing vet to write out the necessary order.

If your pet has a chronic disease, be sure to have whatever will be needed in case of a crisis.

The usual doses

One tablespoon equals 3 teaspoons.

25 drops or 5 milliliters in volume, be it:

    5 grams of water or aqueous solution,

    4 grams of alcohol, or

    6.5 grams of sugar syrup.

One dessertspoon is equal to 2 teaspoons.

One tablespoon equals 3 teaspoons.

One liquor glass is equal to 5 teaspoons, or about 25 grams of water.

One wine glass is equal to 15 teaspoons.

One ordinary glass is about equal to 30 teaspoons, be it:

    150 grams of water,

    120 grams of alcohol or oil, or

    200 grams of sugar syrup.

One handful varies in its equivalent weight according to the grain, running from about 75 grams for light grains to 100 grams for meal.

One meter equals 39.37 inches.

One liter equals 1.06 quarts.

Ten (10) grams equal .35 ounce.

One kilogram equals 2.2 pounds.

To convert from *Centigrade* to Fahrenheit, multiply by $\%$ and add 32°.

Kilo- means 1000; *centi-* means $\frac{1}{100}$; *milli-* means $\frac{1}{1000}$.

► WILD ANIMALS

More and more often these days, especially in rural areas, people have what are called wild animals, some of which are quite easily tamed: the fox, the mongoose, the cheetah, and indeed the tiger and panther (I once had the latter), not to mention monkeys.

Let's not delude ourselves. Despite rare exceptions and even though people pretend to the contrary, animals born free-ranging are never truly comfortable in captivity. For their owners, they are always fascinating, often alarming, and necessarily troublesome. If a cat sharpens his claws on a cushion, it is damaged. If a panther sharpens his claws on a cushion—no more cushion! These excesses can become dangerous, as when a tiger, thinking he's just an overgrown cat, affectionately cuffs you on the shoulder. That once happened to one of my friends. He had to be rushed to the hospital. Furthermore, you might as well know the truth: these animals are invariably dirty. Accustomed to doing his duty anywhere that seems a handy place, a cheetah or fennec can never be trained to go in the street.

There are many kinds of wild animals including primates, canids, felines, marsupials, and rodents.

► PRIMATES

Zaza had the same mischievous eyes as Judith, the famous star of "Daktari" seen on television by the whole world. Like her, she walked on her hind legs, occasionally supporting herself nonchalantly with one of her hands, as if it were a cane. And exactly like Judith, although Zaza loved her master she couldn't resist playing tricks on him in order to get a rise out of him.

Zaza's master and victim was Michel Simon, and she was the apple of his eye for many years. She possessed the astonishing intelligence of chimps, whose capacities sometimes approach man's so closely that it disturbs me.

Zaza had received a radio as a gift from her friend Michel and, just like a real person, she spent hours listening to its sounds. Since this was before the advent of transistors, in order for her to hear these enchanting noises, the radio had to be plugged in. Zaza understood this perfectly well; when she left one room for another, she unplugged the radio and took it with her to plug in elsewhere.

Sometimes the radio went dead. Zaza wouldn't admit that her radio had broken down, and she blamed the socket instead. Scowling, she would pull out the plug and move it somewhere else. Obviously, silence still prevailed. Her eyes clouding over with anger, Zaza would try all of the sockets in the house. Finally, she would have to admit the obvious: the magic music box no longer worked. Possessing a logical mind, Zaza would conclude that she had broken it and so she would try to repair it:

164

first she'd examine it and then, unable to revive it, she'd throw her broken toy angrily to the floor in order to smash it. Wasn't that a very human reaction and wouldn't it have given Voltaire much to philosophize about?

Every day at noon, Zaza sat opposite her human host for lunch. Around her neck was a napkin and in her hand, a fork—a very handy thing, as noblemen of old also knew, for scratching one's back.

When she had had her coffee she yawned, stretched, explained that it was siesta time, and then, having politely excused herself, she left the table and climbed up to her room to rest.

One afternoon Michel Simon, wishing to tell Zaza something, went up to the room where he assumed she was resting. But no ape! He called for her, searched the house, and became alarmed at the thought that she might have run away. He called on neighbors whom he hardly knew, to ask them if by any chance they had seen his chimp.

Then a charming woman opened his door and, before he could speak, she said matter-of-factly:

"Oh, so you were looking for Zaza; well, she just left."

Taken aback, Michel Simon asked, "Was she at your house?"

"Of course. She came just as she does every day, to drink coffee with my husband and me."

Every day? Michel Simon was baffled. Finally, everything became clear.

Several months previously, his neighbors had heard their doorbell ring while having their dessert. They opened their door to find themselves face to face with a big chimpanzee, who held out her hand and apologized for having disturbed them but who obviously hoped that they would invite her in. Greatly amused, they did so. Seeing some coffee, of which she was very fond, Zaza pointed to a cup and explained politely but firmly that if she were offered some, she wouldn't refuse it any more than she would a piece of that cake on the table there.

When Zaza was ready to say good-by, her new friends invited her to return the next day. So she did!

But doubtless fearing that her master would be jealous of them and would forbid her from seeing them, she didn't tell Michel Simon about these visits. At siesta time then, she would climb slowly, sleepily to her room, and as soon as the door was closed, she would climb through the window and over the garden wall, and then call on her neighbors!

You have to hear Michel Simon talk about primates to understand that they can either be admitted to human society, or excluded from it. But you cannot treat them the way you would another animal. It's impossible because they aren't "really" animals. Do you want proof of this? Then consider the fact that the medicine we use to treat them isn't veterinary but human! If you have a primate that needs treatment, I have to direct you to a physician!

All primate therapy, then, is based on the treatment for people. If you have one, treat him like a child; he is a child.

But *don't forget* that since he has the same constitution as a human being, any disease that he gets is contagious for people. And, among other diseases, he is extraordinarily susceptible to tuberculosis.

If a dog or a cat has tuberculosis, it's because he has caught it from a person. But if a primate has it, he has caught it from another primate and can transmit it to a person.

My goddaughter has a monkey that was purchased on a dock. He's a young macaque with grabby hands like a baby, a mischievous look, and lots of energy. She had had him for several days when his bright eyes grew dull and troubled. His look of a child in pain revealed the diagnosis to me.

I was right; he had pneumonia, which appears on x-ray just like human pneumonia.

At the same time as this, my one-year-old nephew also had a similar infection. The illness evolved in the same fashion in the two babies, who were treated exactly alike and recovered at the same time.

Unfortunately, this missing link, although so closely resembling us, is *never* clean, no matter what his species and no matter whether he is big or little. So no matter what you may think, he is not a housepet. Moreover, from any point of view he is a born brat; he breaks things for the fun of it.

One of my friends has a couple of perfectly tame monkeys that roam about freely and whose mischief he ignores because he is as attached to them as he would be to children.

Every Friday the three of them leave by car to spend the

weekend in the country. The macaques, who love to go for a ride, prudently hold onto the armrests.

Some time ago, my friend stopped the car out in the country and went for a walk for a few minutes.

When he returned, no one was in the car. He had forgotten to lock the car; opening it had been a snap—for monkeys!

He called and looked for them everywhere, even ringing the bell of the only house around, and where no one was even living. After an hour, despairing of ever seeing his dear friends again, he decided to start the motor. But at this familiar sound, screeching anxiously to wait for them, the two monkeys jumped down from one of the windows of the farmhouse where he had rung the bell in vain, and got back in the car.

Big hugs, a big hello, apologies all around, everyone was very happy—and my friend found himself covered from head to toe with spots of the most beautiful red color!

Having discovered a jar of paint, the two monkeys had had a delightful time playing painters!

"Then I had some kind of moral lapse," their master admitted to me. "I started the motor and took off at high speed. All of a sudden I had imagined the havoc that they must have caused to the interior of that house. And I thought about how frightened those good folks would be when they returned home to find those red handprints everywhere, left by some horrible demon!"

Personally I would prefer having a lion to a primate; a lion would certainly not be as destructive. But if you don't share my point of view in spite of what I have just said, and you want to own a primate, *don't forget:*

(1) He should be treated, according to his size, as a baby, a child, or an adult.

(2) Ascertain, when you buy him, that he doesn't have tuberculosis: an x-ray is imperative.

(3) Take him for a proctoscopic exam to make sure he doesn't have any parasites. In point of fact, the majority of primates have been captured in the wild and are crammed full—there is no other term—of parasites: coccidia, amebae, lamblia, etc., all *transmissible to man.*

Now I would like to tell you a little anecdote that illustrates my point. Recently I had to operate on a chimpanzee that had broken his femur. I had to get the help of one of my surgeon friends.

When the operation was over, he said to me, somewhat embarrassed:

"I was troubled during the whole procedure by the thought that the man I was operating on was an animal."

I replied, "And I had the same uncomfortable feeling that the animal lying on the operating table was a man!"

CONFINEMENT OF A FEMALE PRIMATE

Several times I have had to attend primates at their deliveries. They actually reproduce quite easily in captivity, especially the smaller species. If you have a pair of monkeys and notice that Mrs. Monkey is in a family way, take care of her the way you would an expectant woman. When the time comes, the delivery will proceed exactly as with a human being.

THE BABY PRIMATE

Mama Monkey may die in bringing her baby into the world. And here you are with a nurseling in your arms—what should you do? Well, proceed just as you would with a human baby.

First of all, put him in swaddling clothes, to replace the missing maternal warmth, and provide a basket and blanket. Then—and this is also urgent—bottle feed. Its contents should be composed of:

about 4 ounces (120 cubic centimeters or milliliters) of cow's milk
about 2 ounces (60 cc.) of water
about ⅓ ounce (10 grams) of honey or sugar.

As soon as you have time, go to the drugstore and buy some baby's milk; it will suit him perfectly. The feeding schedule is the same as that for a human baby, except that a small monkey should imbibe one teaspoonful per suck, and a medium-sized monkey should have the same bottle as a human baby.

I don't think that you'll ever have to raise an orangutan (an endangered species—*Trans.*).

NOTE: When Baby Monkey takes his bottle, hold it vertically until he burps. As you see, there is no difference between him and a human baby, which is why I refer you to any good book on infant care.

HOW TO TELL WHEN A PRIMATE IS SICK

A primate isn't sick just because he sleeps. Even if he sleeps a lot, if he is lively and cheerful when he wakes up, there is nothing to fear.

The two main criteria that allow you to tell when he is in distress are:

(1) lethargy.
(2) a lusterless coat, with lifeless fur.

Last and least, poor appetite. But if a primate has eaten too much the previous evening, he will put himself on a diet the next day; therefore, lack of appetite is only a matter for concern if it is accompanied by the two preceding symptoms.

Constipation

This occurs frequently in primates and makes them irritable. To be healthy, they should have bowel movements just like those of a human being. If you observe that your primate is constipated, treat him as you would yourself.

Diarrhea

When a primate has diarrhea, there is no cause for hesitation: have his stools analyzed immediately, because he may have an intestinal ailment transmissible to man.

Temperature

Body temperature in the great apes resembles that of man and likewise is variable; it is lowest at 5 o'clock in the morning and highest around 5 o'clock in the afternoon. But not everyone owns an orangutan, a gorilla, or even a plain old chimpanzee.

Monkeys, on the other hand, have a much larger deviation between the two circadian extremes: the morning temperature generally ranges from 98.1°F (36.7°C) to 99.5°F (37.4°C), while the evening one varies, according to the species, somewhere between 103.1°F (39.5°C) and 103.6°F (39.8°C). There is one exception: the marmoset's temperature stays at 102.2°F (39°C) 24 hours out of 24.

Of course, as with humans, nervous tension or muscular exertion can cause a rise in temperature.

If primates' temperature resembles that of man very closely, on the other hand it is much more difficult to take than is man's or a dog's or cat's.

Hardly any of them except for chimpanzees accept the thermometer with good grace, and even they must be as well brought up as Judith to do so.

As for the other species, the smaller they are the more they object. Merely seeing the thermometer drives them up a wall, and when a monkey is angry he bites, even if he is the most affectionate thing in the world ordinarily.

If so, there is only one thing to do. If he runs away, he has to be caught with the aid of (according to his size) a butterfly net or a landing net.

Then, while he is still trapped, put on some thick gloves, hold him down within the net with one hand, and take his temperature with the other. But if you have a monkey the size of a macaque, for example, I strongly urge you to wear soldering gloves, the only kind that his sharp teeth won't be able to pierce.

The same advice holds for giving an injection, applying a bandage, etc.

If he lets you handle him, it isn't because he is "gentle" but because he is gravely ill: you should consider him already half dead.

PRIMATE ILLNESSES

Consult a book on child care.

►THE LARGE FELINES

THE LION

One of my friends is the son of a governor-general from colonial times. He once told me this extraordinary story from his childhood.

"I must have been fifteen when a black man brought us a big cat with gentle, innocent, laughing, honey-colored eyes, little round ears, velvet paws, and striking grey-blond fur dotted in light brown. It was a lion cub, several weeks old, whose mother had just been killed.

"We raised him on the bottle and he came to be loved by the whole family.

"He grew up with me and my brothers, always lively, gay, and gentle, and totally oblivious to the fact that he was the king of beasts. One day when we were all in the living room, we heard a lion in love roaring in the distance. Ours perked up his ears, looked at us in obvious fright, and at the next roar dived under a sofa.

"As was readily apparent from his behavior, he assumed himself to be the son of the Great Dane who, although a "dry" nurse, had raised him tenderly and showed no fear of the 330 pounds that he weighed at eight months, giving him a maternal walloping whenever she thought he deserved one.

"Our lion, whom we had christened Titus (he had to have the name of an emperor), was very fond of my father, behind whose bedroom door he wept discreetly when he was forbidden from lying on the bed any more, without even knowing the reason why!

"You could shut all the doors and windows, but when my father went out, Titus would always find a way to jump over a wall and rejoin his person-friend, often interrupting some important official ceremony without any compunctions. When he had finally found his master again, he lay down, purred contentedly at his feet, and didn't budge. My father made him get into the official car to return to the governmental palace, often greatly distressing some local official, for whom our lion courteously saved space next to himself on the seat. I always suspected that my father, who disliked bureaucrats, was just as amused as Titus by the fright that the lion caused them.

"But the inhabitants of the capital themselves became so used to the lion that when they saw him gallop by they no longer even stepped back out of the way. He was simply Monsieur le Gouverneur's lion. . . .

"One day, however, he caused quite a panic in a native village where my father had gone to make a visitation to the chief.

"Right in the middle of the royal meal, all the notables jumped up and fled, screaming in terror: a king of beasts had come into their village! My father had all he could do to prevent the principal hunters from attacking Titus, who was completely baffled by both this headlong flight, which he found very entertaining, and the sharp cries that greeted his appearance, hurting his delicate ears.

"Deeply humiliated, his frightened warriors having made him lose face before the white man whom he suspected of having arranged the incident deliberately, the chief never forgave my father for Titus's impromptu appearance.

"After this episode my father reviewed the positions held by all the members of his staff and, as I had always dreaded he would do, he decreed that at 18 months Titus had become too big to live among people: he had to return to his native forest.

"In funereal silence we had our lion get in the back of the family car, which never bothered him at all; he was so used to it that he rightly considered that that narrow seat belonged to him. Then my father and I, who wanted to stay with Titus up to the final moment, took the road to the forest.

"Having gone what we judged to be a sufficient distance, we made Titus get out of the car and led him toward the forest.

" 'You will see,' said my father optimistically, 'that he recognizes his old habitat and will leave us of his own accord.' "

"I doubt that, in his political affairs, my governor-general of a father was ever so badly mistaken. Titus frolicked about in the thick vegetation, burying himself in it, and we took the opportunity to sneak back into the car. But Titus got in before we did! He had gone for a nice walk and had returned!

"We tried again. This disconcerting game, which Titus found quite amusing, lasted all afternoon.

"At last we succeeded in escaping. We heard a rustling and some indignant roars behind the car.

" 'He'll kill himself trying to follow us,' " I said, grief-stricken. I hated my father! But I half forgave him when I saw that this dignified man was crying like a child.

"Dinner—and no one touched a bite—passed in deathly quiet. Even the servants maintained a reproachful silence.

"At four o'clock in the morning we were all awakened from fitful sleep by roaring beneath our windows: Titus had returned home.

"But he had not seen much humor in the incident. He pouted for several days. Eventually, however, he resumed his life with the family.

"One month later my father decided to try the operation again. We didn't want to sentence Titus to death but even my mother, who adored him, acknowledged that it was difficult, in a place as official as a governor-general's palace, to keep a 550-pound lion who was happily approaching his second birthday.

"I don't know how many times we took Titus out in the forest in order to abandon him, driving farther and farther away each time. He returned so many times, sometimes after having walked for 48 hours.

"Then one day he didn't return. Had he realized that we no longer wanted him?"

But Titus's story doesn't end there. Two years later my friend went on a hunt in the forest, alone. He was 17 years old, the age at which one scorns danger.

Arriving at a clearing, he found himself face to face with a lioness and her two cubs.

"The enraged beast, propelled by muscles as springy and responsive as steel, was already up on her hind legs ready to leap, before I even had time to aim my pistol. But just at that instant, rendering any action on my part impossible, the male surged into view, landing with a fantastic leap between his family and me. I knew that I was finished. But at the same moment I realized that the lion wasn't throwing himself toward me but toward his female, whom he repulsed with blows of his forepaw while roaring some explanation to her.

"Had he ordered her to go away? She withdrew in a huff, followed by her cubs.

"Then the lion turned and bounded up to me, licked my face, and rolled at my feet. I could only murmur, 'Titus! Oh it's you, Titus!' "

"He calmed down, took a few steps toward his wife and children, and turned towards me: he was obviously introducing his family to me.

"He returned to me, licked my hands one more time, and, with supreme dignity, departed, followed by the lioness and cubs.

"For the last time, before re-entering the forest, he turned his head towards me. Then he disappeared. I never saw him again."

Isn't that a wonderful wild animal story? I assure you that it's true.

If you ever have a lion—and you see that this can happen—remember to care for him just like a cat. All you have to do is increase the dosage of medicine you give him. All the same, when he gets somewhat large, I advise you to consult a vet. If you can, choose one who works for a circus or a zoo.

All the other big felines—tigers, panthers, etc.—are cared for like the cat, but of course using larger doses and taking greater precautions. (See the section on Cat care.)

▸ THE CANIDS

THE WOLF

In Morocco I was acquainted with a young wolf. She was four months old and her master, Mr. G., had bought her a month before from a Berber. He brought her to me to have her vaccinated. Like the fox, the wolf is much more subject to distemper than is the dog.

She had the blazing eyes of animals of the apocalypse, but her timid demeanor belied her ferocious look. Gentle and rather passive, she seemed accustomed to her captivity. It is true that, since she was treated as a dog, she never experienced the ignominy of the cage.

Wolf knew and even responded to her name. She sniffed the man's hand affectionately when he came in, and then went to lie down in a dark corner. What was striking about her was that she didn't have the playfulness of young animals; she didn't seem to be familiar with their games.

"Her sadness distresses me," said Mr. G. "But when she was captured, she was hardly two months old. She can't possibly remember that."

One day her master came home and called to her, as was his habit. In vain. The wolf didn't respond to his calls. Unaccountably she had disappeared, as if, like an animal from Hell, she had returned there.

After looking everywhere, he glanced absentmindedly through the window. And he understood what had happened: the body

175

of the little wolf lay four floors below. She had jumped through the window and killed herself.

But why had she jumped, when her instinct for danger must have told her not to?

"She committed suicide," Mr. G. always claimed. "She preferred death to captivity."

Perhaps she had risked everything for the chance to gain her freedom; who can tell?

If you own a wolf or, as is now just as common, a half-wolf (the issue of the mating of a wolf with a dog), care for him exactly as you would a dog. (See the section on Dog care.)

All other canids—foxes, etc.—are cared for like dogs.

‣MUSTELINES AND VIVERRINES

One of my clients recently brought me a very handsome animal resembling, but larger than, a ferret. It was a nandine, one of the tamest of animals.

"She's adorable and affectionate," enthused her mistress. "At night when I go to bed, she jumps up on my bed and goes to sleep against me like a regular little cat. I have brought her to you so you can examine her and tell me how to take care of her."

"Well, first of all, I'm going to vaccinate her against distemper (see *Distemper*, page 73; and *Vaccines*, page 113), since she is a canid."

Several weeks passed and nandine returned with her mistress, who seemed quite upset.

"I don't know what to do," she said. "She's so dirty."

"Yes, unfortunately that is almost always the case with all wild animals, even tame ones. However, usually you can get a nandine to make some effort at cleanliness. Have you tried providing her with a litter box?"

"Like a cat?"

"Of course, since the nandine is a feline."

The young woman looked at me skeptically.

"But Doctor, three weeks ago you told me that she was a canid!"

I realized that my client was wondering what was with this weird vet who changed the classification of animals from week to week. But it wasn't I but rather the nandine which is weird, being both dog and cat at the same time . . . and having the characteristics and the diseases of both!

This being the case, if you have one of these delightful animals, you'll have to care for him as either a feline or a canid, according to what disease he has. The same is true of their brothers and sisters: the mongoose which is also very amiable, the mink, the ferret, the polecat, the skunk, the genet, the civet, the ermine, etc.

▸ RODENTS

THE GUINEA PIG

Originally referred to as the Indian pig, this animal first appeared on tables as a roast, before children made him one of their favorite playthings. Despite his hardy appearance, he is quite delicate and avoids cold and humidity. And despite his last name, he doesn't grunt. On the other hand, never put two males together; they will fight to the death. So if you buy a pair of them, pay close attention to their sexes. But when Madame Guinea Pig has her babies, after 63 days of gestation, she will be able to lie down without fear amid other females, none of whom will act like a witch and kidnap her babies—which is unusual for rodents.

Although larger than hamsters, the guinea pig's life closely resembles that of the hamster (see *The Hamster*, page 180). But the guinea pig doesn't reach adulthood until nine months—although this doesn't prevent him from being extremely precocious in matters of love: he begins mating as early as two months of age, and he has the nerve to keep five females for himself. The guinea pig is a regular rabbit!

Moreover, he is nursed like a rabbit, cared for like a rabbit, and the most serious disease that he can have is, naturally, coccidiosis (see *Coccidiosis*, page 186). But he can also have:

The common cold

The guinea pig can catch colds. He doesn't like the cold and avoids humidity. The least draft starts him sneezing. Treat him with vaseline oil, several drops in each nostril. And put him in a warm place, just as you would any patient with a cold.

Ophthalmia

The guinea pig, like the hamster, can get this. In the latter animal, this condition can progress to the point of drying of the eyeball, but this occurs late in life and cannot be cured. The little guinea pig can, however, be treated. His ophthalmia is actually due usually to a deficiency of vitamin A.

So as soon as you notice that his eyes are red, irritated, and tearing, put him on carrots immediately. As you know, they contain good old vitamin A. You will have no trouble getting him to eat them—he loves them! In addition, wash his eyes every morning and evening with boric acid.

If despite this treatment he doesn't improve, it's because his ophthalmia is due to a streptococcal infection and you'll have to take him to a vet.

Diarrhea

He gets this easily, and more often in spring and summer than in winter, but it isn't serious. He won't die from it; all you have to do is change his diet in order to put everything back in order. Replace his leafy green vegetables with dry feed: crushed oats and bran, and some carrots. Cut down on his water intake and keep him in a warm place, sheltered from drafts, in a box with heavy-duty litter. Everything will return to normal.

THE HAMSTER

Mesocricetus auratus, the little golden hamster, has only lived with man for 45 years. It was in 1930 that Professor Aharoui, a learned English biologist, brought several groups from Syria in order to study the often bizarre behavior of this likeable rodent who, from his head to the tip of his tail, measures less than six inches. The hamster, brought to the banks of the Thames, immediately captivated the English.

This wasn't the first time that this had happened to them. In 1839 Sir Waterhouse, a great adventurer, brought back a specimen that soon won the hearts of all the gentry, who became very fond of the animal.

Alas, after two and a half years the lord's little companion died, to the surprise and chagrin of his human friend, who didn't know that a hamster reaching three years can be considered a centenarian!

But, being a great economizer, this tiny thing who lives such a brief time manages, when out in the wild, to accumulate over 100 pounds (50 kilograms) of provisions! So don't be surprised if you see him store a part of the grain that you offer him in his cage. This doesn't mark a lack of appetite indicating disease, it is simply a fear of scarcity.

Do not worry if you see his cheeks bulge and double in volume: they serve him as both a market basket and a pantry.

Dietary deficiency

If you don't give your hamster the nourishment that he needs, like all rapidly growing animals he will develop a dietary deficiency which can have serious consequences: loss of hair, enteritis, ophthalmia, etc.

If this happens, immediately put him on the highly nutritious diet of rabbits: carrots, cabbage leaves, lettuce, fruit, and of course wheat germ with which he will stuff his jowls, and sunflower seeds which he will husk with his forepaws like a squirrel.

Also add to his food a drop of a multiple vitamin preparation for babies.

Diarrhea in the hamster

If your hamster has diarrhea, it may be due to enteritis caused by a dietary deficiency.

If, however, he is two years old when he gets it, it's due to a streptococcal or staphylococcal infection. In this case, offer him rice water to drink. But have no illusions—this condition will probably spell the end of your little friend.

Reproduction

Miss Hamster was hardly six weeks old when she married Mister Hamster, her senior by three weeks. Then she divorced him, as soon as the marriage had been consummated. A month later, she brought eight tiny babies into the world. Six weeks afterward, her daughters were old enough to get married. She let them live their own lives, and she remarried.

If you are good at math, you can have fun trying to solve the following problem. On January 1 you buy a pair of hamsters. You let them reproduce normally—themselves and their offspring. How many hamsters will you have by December 31 of the same year?

This problem illustrates why you should make sure that Mr. and Mrs. Hamster don't get together too often, at least if you don't want to be invaded by innumerable little rodents. So you'll be much better off with two cages where they can live separately, an arrangement that suits them fine.

Mrs. Hamster has an excuse for her great precocity and her many successive marriages. After one year, she is too old to have children! So of course for the first 12 months she can't waste any time.

As soon as she becomes pregnant, provide scraps of cotton rags and wool from which she can make her nest and thus keep her litter warm, for the young come into the world completely hairless. They have to wait two weeks before they get their fur coats.

Then let nature take her course. Everything will go well if you don't interfere.

Sleep in a hamster

One day, a curious adventure happened to one of my actress friends, who was as famous as she was beautiful.

During the Algerian crisis I opened an evening newspaper and saw her photo on the first page. Considering her renown, I wasn't very surprised at first—but she wasn't being mentioned in regard to any film. She had just been arrested as a dangerous agent of the Secret Army Organization.

Some friendly, patriotic, and curious neighbors had denounced her to the police for clandestine broadcasting.

"Every night we have heard her sending out messages in Morse code," they had testified categorically.

I was astonished. My lovely friend had never been concerned with political matters in her whole life. She even made fun of such concerns. Yes . . . but on the other hand, she adored hamsters—which were what the police who came to search her house found instead of a transmitting station.

Hamsters have a peculiarity: they sleep all day and are active at night. As soon as night fell and they were wide awake, the five or six that she owned gnawed, ate, and played to their hearts' content.

It was these unusual noises that the worried neighbors had heard and had mistaken for clandestine broadcasts!

I relate this little anecdote in order to remind you of this peculiarity of hamsters, which is nothing to be interfered with, at least if you don't want to see them waste away and quickly die.

If you have children as well as hamsters, as is generally the case, you should teach them this: they should never, either to play with their hamsters or even to pet them, awaken them while they are asleep during the day.

THE RABBIT

I know a completely tame and highly civilized rabbit who gets walked on a leash, travels by car, and nestles on his owner's knees to munch carrots.

This rabbit is so well off and so sure of himself that he has become aggressive. Recently his owner brought him to me to be vaccinated against rabies; the two of them had to go on a trip. In my office I had a pleasant German shepherd who glanced indifferently at what he took to be a harmless rodent, when suddenly the little thing transformed itself into some kind of prehistoric monster and threw itself on the dog with the obvious intention of putting him out of commission permanently. The poor dog, who had never had a rabbit charge him before, ran away barking in terror. This seemed to gratify Jeannot's master quite a bit; he said to me, not without pride:

"He can't abide German shepherds."

That was obvious.

I bring this up to make note of the fact that a rabbit who doesn't know how man has treated his brethren under most circumstances can be a very good friend to him and can be tamed as well as any domestic animal and exhibit gentleness or even a nasty disposition. Several of my patients are rabbits.

Rabbits captured as babies and raised like kittens are as tame and gentle as cats. So it is quite possible that you will own one some day. If so, you should know one thing right off:

You don't have to stop him from eating his feces. They are essential for him.

One of my clients is a model, a very beautiful girl who has a darling Angora—not a cat but a rabbit. The first time she brought him to me was because he was a skeleton.

"But God knows he eats," she said to me. "Lettuce, cabbage, everything—he doesn't stop. I go to the market every morning for him."

"What do you do with his excrement?" I asked her.

"Oh, I dispose of it at once; what do you think?"

"Well, you shouldn't be surprised that your rabbit is in the process of slowly dying from hunger. And you could give him all the cabbage in the world and you wouldn't stop it. You have to let him eat his feces or at least part of them."

Gnawing animals actually have two types of excrement: nocturnal and diurnal. The nocturnal type is the product of an initial predigestion, so the animal has to eat it again to sustain himself. This is what enables these animals to nourish themselves as well on a piece of wood as on a carrot.

This predigestion is their way of preparing their meals internally. The initial digestive product, which is always soft, constitutes a well-prepared entree that nourishes them. On the other hand, they never consume the second, hard excretory product; they deposit it properly in a corner.

This is the most important thing to remember about rabbits. But, like all other animals, they can get sick.

(The rabbit technically is not a rodent, but a lagomorph— *Trans.*)

Coenurosis

This has exactly the same cause as cysticercosis, but the larvae remain in the intestine.

Cysticercosis

One of my clients had a Skye terrier—you know, one of those dogs with long hair and short legs so that everything gets tangled up together but all the while the dog maintains a very British dignity. One morning she brought the dog an adorable little blue-grey, long-haired ball as a present. The Skye terrier's heart swelled at this sight and, filled with motherly love, she took the little thing in her paws and at once began to wash it intensely. The grey ball sniffed a little but didn't protest. This was the start of a great friendship.

But Miss Skye Terrier had been fooled: this wasn't a baby dog but rather a baby Angora rabbit. Older matrons do sometimes fail to make these distinctions.

This is to emphasize that a dog and rabbit raised together get along very well. However, the dog can present a mortal danger to his friend if he is unlucky enough to have tenia. This is a vicious circle because initially it is the rabbit, debilitated by the disease, who frequently communicates the tenia to the dog. (See *Tenia*, page 114.)

Obviously this process is reversible also.

One morning you notice that the little animal has bumps under his skin: cysts caused by the larvae of the worm. These can kill him so, if you are attached to your rabbit, you'll have to think about deworming your dog. It is better still to deworm both animals; the rabbit can himself transmit these parasites to his friend.

Coccidiosis

This is sometimes popularly referred to as "big belly." It is very serious because it can lead to death. These protozoans are transmitted when the rabbit eats very fresh, overly watery vegetables. Consult the vet at once; only he can save your pet.

NOTE: If your rabbit has a mate, immediately separate her from the male and disinfect their abode with *a soldering lamp* before putting them back in: nothing is more contagious than coccidiosis. Do the same thing for guinea pigs (see *The Guinea Pig*, page 179).

Itchy ears

This is treated just as it is in the cat or dog. (See *Itchy ears*, page 84.)

Poisonous plants

If you have a rabbit and are going to the country, you will surely bring him back some plants as a treat.

NOTE: Many plants are poisonous and some are fatal for your lagomorph friend: blue or scarlet pimpernel, anemone, aconite, hemlock, belladonna, meadow saffron, foxglove, mustard, poppy, primula, ranunculus (buttercup), and St. John's wort. Lastly, if your rabbit is a female who is nursing babies, don't give her parsley or chervil, which may "cut" her milk.

Myxomatosis

Fatal to rabbits, this condition is the province solely of vets. You may be able to recognize it by the presence of soft tumors in the body.

If your rabbit has myxomatosis, you may be required to report the case to health authorities.

Vaccines

If you have a female rabbit and you decide to let her have young, don't forget one very important thing: have her vaccinated before and during pregnancy. You thus assure her babies the maximum chance of survival.

Preventive vaccinations

These should take place four times per year and are different each time since rabbit diseases are seasonal. If you have a tame rabbit, and especially if you ever take him out into the country, these vaccinations are absolutely essential. Don't forget that certain fatal diseases, such as myxomatosis, are transmitted by flies.

Beginning from the 25th day of life, the rabbit should receive the following vaccinations every year:

spring: enterotoxemia
summer: myxomatosis
fall: pasturellosis (pulmonary infection)
winter: mucoid enteritis

THE WHITE RAT

I won't discuss the brown rat or the grey rat; these animals should never be tamed because they are the most formidable carriers of disease: typhus, leptospirosis, and others.

The white rat, however, can make an agreeable and very intelligent companion. Raise him like a rabbit (see *The Rabbit*, page 183); the only difference is that he is an omnivore and will never turn down beef. I warn you that, like all wild animals, rats in cages often kill their young.

THE WHITE MOUSE

One day a very interesting thing happened to one of my clients. She owned a Burmese cat who tried to hunt mice. Also living in the house, but duly separated from the cat, was a pair of white mice which belonged to her ten-year-old son.

These charming rodents have babies every two months, five or six per litter which, from the age of five weeks, are eager to mate in their turn. Make a rough guess as to how many of them Mrs. D. found when she entered her son's room. It was enough to scare any woman, even one not frightened by the sight of a mouse's tail!

What to do? Mrs. D. thought about the situation and then made a tragic decision. While her little boy was at school, she set the white mice free after having let her Burmese cat into the room.

Then she went out, not wanting to witness the horrible spectacle. She took ten steps away from the house but, torn by remorse and feeling like a murderess, she ran back inside to stop the slaughter—if there was still time!

How many survivors would she find?

She pushed open the door of the room, not daring to look, her heart beating wildly. She glanced out furtively and then opened her eyes wide. Lying on his back and purring, his four paws in the air, the Burmese was playing the role of Gulliver in the land of the dwarfs. Without any fear or uneasiness, the mice were tickling his stomach and armpits, making him squirm with delight. One of them was delicately curled up in his thick tail, another nibbled at his ear.

The cat had a look full of indulgence on his face. He turned to his mistress as if to say that these were "his" mice and the dear little things were having so much fun that he had to let them play—at cat and mouse!

If you have white mice and don't want to find yourself in the same predicament as Mrs. D., you see that you can't trust a housecat to control the situation. So separate the males from the females at birth. You can identify the males at once: they immediately begin to fight among themselves. I suggest that you do the same with white rats, even though they are less prolific.

The diseases of these rodents are fairly uncommon occurrences and are treated like those of hamsters (see *The Hamster*, page 180) or guinea pigs (see *The Guinea Pig*, page 179).

► THE HORSE

I know the horse well since for several years I took care of
the breeding stud of the king of Morocco.

One thing should be clarified right away: with all such "big
animals," the vet is much more qualified than you to take care of
them, at least if you are not a "horseman" but only a "regular"
man. And there is quite a bit that horsemen don't know about.

Therefore I'll only discuss "emergencies" here—cases in which
you are very far from a vet and only the alacrity of your response
can save your animal.

The horse was introduced to the civilized world by the Cretans
about 5000 years ago. But he is no longer that "noble conquest"
that allowed man to explore and settle over long distances for so
much of history. Today, replaced by invisible horsepower, he is
barely a shadow of his former self. The military, of which he was
the pride and joy, has abandoned him.

Alas, for the horse, the vet alone is not enough. Another man
must be at his side, without whom nothing would be possible:
the blacksmith.

If the horse no longer occupies first place on the functional
level, he still is important—in some respects more and more so—
to the life of modern man. He remains indispensable, obviously,
in herding cattle and other large livestock. On racetracks
throughout the world he is a living lottery ticket for bettors. And
he is a source of joy for everyone who loves him for himself and
not for what he can bring them.

Young people everywhere are rediscovering him. He is a delightful traveling companion who provides them with the pure pleasure of tranquil rides through fields and forests.

Almost all rural resorts now have riding schools and horses to ride. Young people can thus become acquainted with the "noblest conquest of man." Moreover, I know more and more horsemen who have built stables next to their garages. In writing that which follows, I was thinking particularly about such horse owners as these—full of affection for their animals but also of inexperience.

HOW TO BUY A HORSE

If, having never had a horse, you decide to buy one, you have three alternatives. Whichever you choose, if you are a novice, I suggest that you take a vet or a horseman along with you.

The animal can be purchased:

From a breeder: You can be certain of the quality of your animal but don't have any illusions about the price: it will be in relation to the quality!

At a racetrack: At the end of Claiming Races, the competing horses are sold. In France, the price schedule is rather curious. At the start of the race, the owners declare their prices. But the horse that comes in first is sold at double this figure! The prices of the other horses, regardless of how they finish, don't change, unless competitive bidding opens.

At the knife: This rather surprising term means that you buy a slaughterhouse horse. It is by far the easiest solution; it doesn't prevent you from having a very handsome animal that you will love all the more because you saved his life.

In any event, a horse can be returned after purchase, if you notice that he has a redhibitory defect or a contagious disease.

REDHIBITORY DEFECTS

These are chronic diseases or defects that legally permit a buyer to return a horse. The law varies on these, so consult a local vet as soon as you detect any abnormality in your new horse. Here are some typical defects in horses:

(1) *Asthma or pulmonary emphysema:* irregular respiration rendered visible by movements of the flanks. Expiration is effected in two steps.

(2) *Lameness:* a type of lameness, which comes and goes with changes in temperature—after a workout or in leaving the stable —may be covered by law.

(3) *Chronic wheezing:* after having trotted or galloped, the horse, when he breathes, emits a sort of snort but exhibits no other signs of respiratory disease.

(4) *Periodic inflammation of the eyes:* this is an intermittent disease manifested by redness, tearing, and a flaky white deposit on the eyeball.

(5) *Immobility:* this is a permanent diminution of the horse's motor function. The animal actually goes crazy. He stands there without budging, too stupid to eat his hay, as if he had forgotten how to swallow!

(6) *Tic:* with or without worn down teeth. The horse actually has aerophagia, which makes him belch conspicuously. Particularly when he is eating, he takes in air and this impedes his swallowing. In addition, he may habitually press his teeth against his feeding crib and wear them down.

(7) *Certain contagious diseases* may be covered by law: glanders, mange, and some diseases that have almost totally disappeared: dourine, pernicious anemia, anthrax, farcy, and rabies.

HOW TO CARE FOR A HORSE

Handling a horse

Several years ago I entered the stall of a sick horse and left the stall much more rapidly than I had gone in—and I found myself confined to a bed for 25 days!

I had thought that the owner, who called himself a "horseman," had "gentled" the animal. But he wasn't gentle at all and, being irritable because of his discomfort, he greeted me with a kick in the stomach!

Thus, one of the most important things to do *while waiting for the vet* is to *gentle* your horse so he doesn't injure the doctor who has come to take care of him.

Moreover, if instead of a vet it is you who are treating him, the same precautions should be taken.

Handling an animal that weighs around 900 pounds (400 kilograms) isn't the same as for a 1-ounce canary. It calls for a whole rigmarole: twitch, halter, leading-rein.

Proceed by:

(1) *Feeding:* Never give a horse who has to be examined anything to eat, because he hates being disturbed during a meal. He demonstrates his bad mood with a swift kick at whoever interrupts his repast—one never knows when one's oats are going to be stolen!

(2) *The halter:* This is used to take the horse out of the stable. The vet can examine him much better and more safely outside. The principle is the same as for light shined in a cat's eyes (see *How To Care for a Cat,* page 120).

(3) *Raising a foreleg:* This means raising either front hoof. The horse thus finds himself on three legs, off balance; hence he cannot kick.

If the horse is rambunctious, keep him steady by using a whip in addition; merely threatening with the whip can be sufficient.

(4) *The twitch:* an instrument of mild punishment that consists of a tube of wood about 20 inches (50 centimeters) long, equipped with a ring at one end. A thong is passed through the ring and the two ends are tied together. Loop the thong around the horse's nose and rotate the stick so as to twist the thong.

The horse's nose thus gets squeezed in the loop and the more that you tighten it, the more you hurt him. He actually has a very sensitive cartilagenous structure between the two nasal bones.

The animal is so distracted by this pain that he can be examined without reacting.

Instead of squeezing the nose, apply pressure to the ear in the same fashion; it too is very sensitive.

(5) *The leading-rein:* If the horse is very skittish or if you are examining the ano-genital or rectal area (the vet can probe sometimes as far as the liver in a rectal examination), you need to use a leading-rein.

The leading-rein is made up of a long rope which has a good stretch of braid and a ring at the end. Pass the end of the rope through the ring and tie the free end around the horse's hind leg above the hoof. The rope is drawn under the arse (the underside of the horse, spanned by drawing the rope between the two forelegs), and you find yourself standing in front of the animal and holding the large loop formed by the braid. Slip the loop over the horse's head (the rope is braided so as not to injure the neck—which a rope would certainly do). Obviously, if the horse tries to kick, he pulls on the rope and thus tightens the slip knot that encircles his neck. Since he doesn't want to strangle himself, he cuts this movement short at once. Thus you can be sure that you won't be kicked.

When the horse has a leading-rein plus a twitch plus a raised foreleg, you can make him undergo anything; he is reduced to complete immobility. And how very important it is for a vet to know how to do this, I assure you!

Lastly, if a drug must be swallowed or the mouth examined, a gag is also needed so that you can keep his mouth open without getting bitten.

HOW TO ADMINISTER A DRUG

By mouth: Obviously this isn't a matter of opening the mouth by hand to get the pill swallowed. A horse isn't a "nice bow-wow."

If he must swallow a pill, use a horse's gag; that is, a buccal speculum, of which several varieties exist. So:

(1) Make the horse hold still in the manner described above.
(2) Open his mouth and keep it open by means of the above-mentioned gag.
(3) Pull the horse's tongue over to one side.
(4) Slip the drug behind the tongue.

Medicine for horses to take by mouth is supplied in the form of an enormous pill, the size of a small ball.

If a liquid drug is prescribed:

(1) Steady the horse as indicated previously.

(2) Fill a bottle with the medicine.

(3) Wrap a rag around the neck of the bottle so that it doesn't cut the horse's mouth.

(4) Insert the bottle neck into the horse's lips, between the cheek and the teeth. NOTE: Never open his mouth in order to get him to drink, as the liquid may go down the wrong pipe.

(5) Raise up the horse's head and let the liquid run down.

By injection: see *Injections* in Horses, page 220.

By enema: Use an enema and a rubber tube that you introduce into the rectum a good 8 inches (20 centimeters). There is nothing more to it than to lift the enema up above the horse by the same distance.

FIXATION ABSCESS

In a desperate case you can try to form an artificial abscess as you can in a dog (see *Fixation Abscess,* page 10). To do so, inject 10 cubic centimeters of turpentine. His 900 pounds will easily sustain such a dose sufficient "to choke a horse."

The injection is made on either side of the median line of the horse's chest (2 inches or 5 centimeters to either side), at the spot where the pectoral muscles begin.

FOALING

I was a vet fresh out of school when I had to deliver my first foal, in Berlin. Up until then, I had only considered the process in theory.

Anyway, when that German mare saw me appear, she stopped her delivery cold. She stood right up: the horse is the only animal that can voluntarily delay delivery. So this event, which unsettled me greatly, was in fact perfectly normal: Mrs. Mare is very modest and refuses to show the light of day to her foal in the presence of a human being.

This rule is so categorical that when I was the veterinarian of King Hassan II, I had a room with a viewing window built adjacent to the "lying-in hospital"; this allowed me to observe deliveries without the animal's seeing or even smelling me.

I mention this so that, if your mare is at term, you are aware that she must not detect your presence. Manage it however you can, but observe her with the utmost discretion.

Moreover, the mare delivers her young very well by herself and with an extraordinary rapidity: it usually takes no more than 20 minutes. (Prey species cannot afford the heightened risk of predation entailed in lengthy periods of vulnerability; toward this same end, their young are "precocial": able to flee with the herd shortly after birth.—*Trans.*)

If by chance there are difficulties, they are very serious and call for a vet's expertise. While waiting, don't pull on the foal because its doctor will probably want to push it back in so as to change its presentation. Above all, don't do what one of my clients did, which I'll never forget: observing that Baby Colt was poorly positioned, he tied a rope around its legs, which were already out, and attached it to a pulley—and pulled! The foal certainly came out—along with the mother's insides. When I arrived, I recognized the disaster that had taken place but couldn't apply any remedy.

Be advised also that:

The mare has a gestation period of 11 months. Breeders say precisely 11 months and 11 days, plus one day for each year of age.

Once she has delivered her foal, she is receptive to being approached.

NOTE: The following day, however, she will be ferocious and will no longer tolerate your presence.

Take advantage of her temporary good disposition to wash and disinfect her with a solution of 2% permanganate. Then tie the umbilical cord and administer first aid, as necessary, as you would for the birth of a puppy (see *Delivering Pups,* page 15).

ACROBYSTITIS

There is a touching story about a lord and a peasant maiden, but alas, like many love stories, it has a sad ending.

"Lord" was a marvelous thoroughbred whose ancestry on both sides could be traced back to the days of chivalry. And he grazed on the greenest pastureland in all of Normandy.

In the neighboring prairie, which was just as green but had grass that was a little less refined, a young donkey dreamed of her prince charming. It must be said that with her soft grey coat and with eyes that seemed to be gazing at the infant Jesus, she was beautiful.

Lord noticed her.

As for her, she had been in love with him for a long time.

One day he jumped over the hedge that separated them and he joined her.

And I received a telephone call from her frightened owner:

"Lord can't piss any more," he informed me rather directly. "Please come right away."

I came. Being a horseman, he had gentled Lord as I have described (see *Handling a horse,* page 191), and I only had to examine him. I found that his sheath was very inflamed.

"Has he by any chance had some amorous adventures lately?"

"Well . . . that is, I did come across the animal while he was covering the farmer's donkey."

I began to laugh.

"You needn't search any further: the donkey was too narrow for him and this chafed him—that's the cause of all his problems. It's not serious."

I prepared some warm cresol solution, one part per thousand, and washed the penis externally with it. Then, using a 3-quart (3-liter) enema, I gave it an injection.

Cresol is a horse's friend. This is the only way to cure this venereal disease rapidly, which is quite common in stallions. I know what I'm talking about because I've seen many a case.

INJURED JOINT

As I have said, cresol, like blue vitriol, is a horse's friend. You should always keep a bottle in your equine medicine chest—you'll haul it out more than once a year. If your animal injures a joint, reach for this bottle first in order to disinfect the wound.

To do so, prepare a warm 3% solution (30 cubic centimeters per liter—about a quart—of water) and wash the sore with it.

Then apply some ether or iodoform. Next apply a dry dressing, consisting of cotton and a tight bandage.

After completing these initial steps, see the vet.

BRUISES

These are contusions, with or without an open sore, of the pastern, the coronet, or the talon: these three parts constitute the upper part of the horse's foot.

Often, it's the horse's neighbor that is responsible for his bruises—horses can "kick like a horse"! A horse frequently bruises himself. When trotting, for example, he often injures his foreleg with the shoe of a hind leg.

Wash and disinfect the wound (always with our 3% cresol solution). Then, most important of all, take the horse to the blacksmith right away because the problem is really one of farriery.

INJURED BARS

As you may know, the bars are the part of the horse's mouth where there aren't teeth and where the bit goes. Some riders, who are either cruel or lacking in experience, pull too hard on the bit and injure the horse.

This condition becomes apparent when the horse drools a lot and also shies away when you try to insert the bit, because it hurts him.

You must then:

(1) Avoid using the bridle until the wound is healed.

(2) Disinfect it with a common disinfectant (cresol at 1 part per thousand, ether, hydrogen peroxide, etc.).

(3) Give a liquid diet—what is referred to by the term mash. I follow the English method of preparation:

1 dry quart (roughly 1 liter) of barley meal
2 quarts of oats.
Add 3 quarts (about 3 liters) of boiling water, and then add 3 dry quarts of bran.

Let stand all day; the pail should be covered with a cotton rag to retard cooling and evaporation of this "soup."

In the evening, stir the mixture with a wooden spatula and serve the still-warm mash to the horse—who will love it.

NOTE: Some equine gourmands gobble down this delectable meal too quickly. If this happens, add two or three quarts of chopped straw to the boiled mixture; this will force the animal to stretch out his gastronomic enjoyment.

HARNESS WOUNDS

These are usually caused by saddles, breast-collars, or bridles that are too hard or too tight. They can also result from the fact that the horse is skinny. In such a case, the withers protrude and the harness rubs against and injures them.

Mole

Let's review a little equine anatomy. The horse's head, which is very heavy, is attached to the body by a very large ligament, the cervical ligament, which runs between the occiput and the withers.

When harnessing the horse, it is obvious that the bridle or halter rests just on the occiput. If there is a defect in saddlery so that the horse is injured at this spot, it's called a mole. It can be inconsequential but it can also be very severe since it can develop into "necrosis of the ligament." Naturally this complication is not within the owner's province—but it is up to him to prevent it. As soon as he notices that the animal's hair is worn away at that spot, he should immediately go to see the harnessmaker.

Neck sores

These are caused by a breast-collar or other collar that fits too tightly.

Withers sores

These are caused by the strap of the horse blanket or by the saddle, especially a sidesaddle, which rubs more on one side than the other. If the horse is just a little thin, this is enough to produce a sore.

Kidney sores

This is also due to a saddle that is too hard.

For all of these, preventive treatment consists of good saddlery.

Similarly, curative treatment is a matter of saddlery; the harness has to be adjusted so as not to injure the animal.

But remedial care is also involved:

(1) Remove the harness from the horse and don't put it on again until he is completely healed.

(2) Hose down the animal with cold water (a garden hose works very well).

(3) Apply an astringent. To do so, make up equal parts of:

powdered chalk
clay
vinegar

If the wound causes an abscess, apply hot flaxseed poultices to accelerate the healing process. The matter will then be up to the vet.

LIMPING

If a horse limps, you have to determine first of all which foot he is favoring, so that you can inform the vet. As important as this is to know, it is just as difficult to determine, and usually one is fooled!

There is, however, a way of finding out: by looking at the head and especially the head and neck together, which horsemen refer to as the balance.

If the horse is favoring a foreleg, he will turn his head and let his neck fall, when he walks, toward the side of the healthy leg. There is no mistaking this; he does it so as to free the affected leg of some of the weight of the balance.

If he favors a hind leg, he holds his head toward the affected side but to a lesser extent, since comparatively little weight is removed by this adjustment.

You then need to determine what is causing the limp. To do so, walk the horse on hard ground and then on soft ground.

If he limps more on hard ground, the limp is caused by bone damage (usually osteitis of the third phalanx).

If the limp is more accentuated on soft ground, the problem is with a tendon.

Inform the vet of your findings when he arrives.

BOULET (Misaligned Fetlock-Joint)

It was in Morocco; I had just made a 20-mile trip when, returning to the stable, I noticed that my horse's fetlock-joints were very swollen.

As you may know, the fetlock-joint is located between the pastern and the cannon bone.

The deformity that I had just detected is called boulet, and it is caused by faulty shoeing.

My horse had been shod with his talons too high, so he was too upright. After the long ride that I had imposed on him, his tendons were fatigued and this led to the inflammation.

I didn't hesitate. I grabbed the garden hose and hosed his legs down until it was I who was fatigued. He enjoyed every minute of it.

Then I let him rest and went to find my blacksmith. The healing of the boulet now depended on his skill.

That is exactly what you should do in a similar situation (see also *Injuries*, page 218).

NOTE: Untreated boulet can be serious and even disastrous.

BRONCHITIS

If your horse coughs, if he has difficulty breathing, he has bronchitis.

You'll have to call the vet but while you're waiting:

(1) Take the animal's temperature (see *Temperature,* page 226; that will give you an accurate indication.

(2) Apply hot mustard plasters. This ancient remedy works wonderfully on a horse.

The mustard plaster should be proportional to the great size of his thoracic cage. Use big pieces of an old sheet and 5 or 6 pounds (2-3 kilograms) of powdered mustard that you dilute in very hot water until you obtain a thick pulp.

(3) Fumigate the patient!

To do so, pour several quarts (liters) of boiling water into a tub, along with 5 or 6 tablespoons of an emollient with a eucalyptus base. Then shut the horse in the horse-box along with the basin.

If you don't have any eucalyptus on hand, use old-fashioned "hay water." Prepare it by throwing 2-4 pounds (about 1-2 kilograms) of chopped hay into some boiling water. If you have some, add 2-3 tablespoons of creosote (distilled from wood tar).

BURNS

When I was a child spending my vacations in Sologne, one of those minor events took place which, when one is 12 years old, take on monumental significance.

My friends were the baker and his horse. The baker had a big white apron and his hands were white with flour. The horse was a fine Percheron, atop which the man's floury hands would set me.

One night I was awakened by shouting. A glimmer of light filled my room as if dawn were breaking. I ran to the window. Right in front of me, glistening from the pailfuls of water that the villagers, forming a bucket brigade, were throwing on it, the baker's barn burned.

In that barn my friend lived.

My heart skipped a beat and, in my pajamas, my hair all mussed up and my eyes swollen first by sleep and then by tears, I hurried outside with but one thought in mind: to save my pal from the same fate as that of Joan of Arc.

Pushed aside by the big people who didn't want to stumble over a little kid, I succeeded nevertheless in getting up to the barn—just in time to see the baker and his horse come out. Alas, just as they came through the door a blazing beam fell on my four-legged friend, burning him grievously.

I cried so loudly that the good man came up to me. With his hands, which were all black that evening, he patted my cheeks:

"Don't be afraid, my boy. I'll be able to cure your horse. Come on, we're going to take care of him together."

And, abandoning his barn which was eventually completely consumed, he led the animal, neighing in pain, toward his house. Several minutes later he applied a compress, smeared with some mysterious liquid, to the horse's wounded rump. As if by magic, it seemed to me, the animal stopped neighing. About a week later, even though the burn had been deep, nothing remained of it but a scar.

As I found out afterwards, that remarkable elixer was none other than my trusty oleocalcareous liniment for which I have already given you the recipe (see *Burns* in Dogs, page 36). It must be said that it works extremely well on horses.

Similarly, when horses are burned, they are treated in general exactly as dogs are. (See *Burns* again.)

Burns with open sores

When burns cause open sores, they absolutely must not be treated with irritating antiseptics. The best way to treat them is the following:

(1) Wash them with a solution of either 10% boric acid or 1% cresol.

(2) Pour over the wounds a mixture of equal parts:

vegetable oil
oil of turpentine
⅕ carbon disulfide (carbon disulfide is found in all drug-stores).

But if you cannot find these, there is always:

The colonel's recipe

When I was a young veterinarian in the army, I had a colonel. He was an old veteran if ever there was one, born in the saddle, as knowledgeable about horses as anyone, but as ornery as he was smart—which was saying a lot.

One day when I asked him for some drugs for my horses, he foamed with rage. Like himself, they should be treated "without" medicine! And he immediately gave me an illustration.

"When I had some burned horses in Syria" (burned in warfare, apparently), "I had nothing available, but I healed some holes as big as my kepi by filling them with lochia oil!" (He had a rather small head, it should be noted.)

I paid respectful attention while suppressing a half-skeptical, half-amused smile.

Then one day, way out in the bush country, I had to treat a burned horse. Having nothing else available, I tried my colonel's lochia oil.

Well, the old buzzard had been right! Particularly in very hot regions, lochia oil repels first flies and later microbes—none of them can survive it. This therefore allows healing to take place without infection.

Anyway, my colonel was only resurrecting a drug employed by the Indians in olden days. In an age when naphtha had not yet become gasoline, they used it to treat their horses' wounds!

BROKEN-KNEED HORSE

You have doubtless often come across a horse wearing a leather knee-piece—he's broken-kneed. This is a knee injury that isn't very serious and is almost always due to a fall.

However, it often indicates that the animal has a bad master. It frequently occurs at small riding stables where the horses are mistreated.

I have seen it in Tunisia. The director of one of these joints had his horses ridden around a corral for five hours and then taken on two long rides every day. The animals, of course, got worn out, and each evening one of them was broken-kneed.

So I implore you, acknowledge that your noblest conquest has a right, just as you do, to rest—even though he isn't unionized. Don't make him exert himself beyond his capabilities!

However, even a contented horse can stumble on a sharp rock and become broken-kneed. So here is how to treat this condition:

(1) Wash the wound with a 10% solution of zinc chloride which the druggist will prepare for you. If for any reason you can't get some, use whatever disinfectant is available (see *Open Wounds*, page 221).

(2) Paint the area with camphorated naphthol (which you can get at a pharmacy), or else with iodized alcohol or with mercurochrome.

(3) Apply a somewhat tight bandage: cotton held in place with an elastic bandage and a leather knee-pad (which you can get at a blacksmith's).

NOTE: If you have a sporting horse that runs obstacle courses, he can very easily hit a barrier and get this condition, especially in the trave.

PAVEMENT NAIL SORE

This appellation dates back to the first studded pedestrian crossings. At some time or another, one of those big nails came loose and, with a bit of bad luck, turned upside down so the point was in the air.

During that period there were still quite a few horse-drawn delivery wagons. If one of these horses had the misfortune to step on the point, he buried it in his hoof.

Deliveries in Paris are no longer made with horses, but the term still remains for all puncture wounds caused by big nails, pebbles, or pieces of broken glass that horses get embedded in their "soles." Such a case is a problem for a blacksmith, since the hoof has to be scraped. But while you are waiting for him:

(1) Withdraw whatever is embedded in the foot.

(2) Let the horse rest because the condition obviously is very painful.

(3) Wash the wound immediately with a hot 10% cresol solution.

(4) Don't forget to "gentle" the horse for the vet's visit (see *Handling a horse,* page 191). If you don't, the vet won't catch pavement nail-sore, but he may get a swift kick which will put him in bed for three weeks! The noblest conquest of man isn't all that friendly when he is in pain.

SWOLLEN PHARYNGEAL POUCHES

It often happens, following a throat infection for example, that a horse develops an accumulation of pus inside the Eustachean tubes. It appears as a very large, soft swelling that can be felt behind the ear. The horse also has trouble breathing and swallowing.

I mention this because it is a malady peculiar to horses. However, it is exclusively a matter for the vet to handle.

COLIC

In May of 1961, when I was employed by the king of Morocco, I was awakened one night by one of the stud horse's grooms. One of Hassan II's handsomest horses was colicky. This is extremely serious in a horse, and if it isn't taken care of in time, it can be fatal.

So I got up in a hurry and went to the stables.

About 45 minutes later, having finished with the horse, I returned to bed at last, slid under the warm covers, and someone again knocked on my door—a second horse had colic.

I ran back to the stable, took care of him, and returned. Then a third horse was stricken with abdominal pain; at least this time I was spared the trouble of returning to my bed.

This was already quite astonishing, for there was no epidemic of colic. But what followed was even more amazing: all twelve of the stud's mares got colic that same night!

Dead tired after eight hours without sleep, obsessed by a situation that I had never encountered before, at dawn I summoned a servant to bring me a large breakfast, which I really needed. Instead, a terrified Berber came and told me:

"The city of Agadir no longer exists!"

"What?" I didn't understand.

"Turn on the radio, Doc; you'll hear about it."

It was the tragic night when Agadir was completely destroyed by an earthquake.

None of the people in Rabat had felt anything—the horses had! More sensitive than a seismograph, they had felt that terrifying force 400 miles away, and their fear had started their intestines in motion!

This painful and serious malady can actually have several causes, one of which is fright.

You can tell that a horse has colic because he paws the ground with his forelegs and turns about in agitation. I have even seen them sit down on their rear ends like Walt Disney's animals and cry like babies because the pain was so bad. But the most important sign of all is that the horse himself will show you what hurts him by turning his head toward his flank. If the colic is caused by his liver, he will point to his liver with his nose. And if the origin is his colon, he will turn his head to the right. He couldn't possibly be any clearer, and if you don't understand, it is you who are the dumb animal!

The horse has several types of colic:

Nervous colic, such as that caused by the Agadir earthquake.

Colic of pregnant mares.

Sand colic, caused by swallowing sand.

Hepatic colic.

Nephritic colic, due to kidney stones, some of which are very large.

Colic due to intestinal congestion. These cases are usually the most serious. Once I saw an autopsy of a horse that died of intestinal obstruction: between the mucosa and the serosa there were 6 inches (15 centimeters) of blood!

Colic due to indigestion or to intestinal occlusion.
Colic caused by intestinal worms, if the animal has been poorly de-wormed.
Colic due to the cold.
The gripes (see *The Gripes,* page 228).

Treatment, therefore, varies greatly according to the syndrome, but whatever the case is, while you wait for the vet:

(1) Never allow the animal to lie down: a horse that lies down is a horse resigned to death.

(2) Put a blanket over him and keep walking him, in order to try to get his intestine to work.

(3) If you are sure that it's due to the cold, have him swallow a good-sized glass of ether (see *How to Administer a Drug,* page 193). This will calm and soothe him. It can also be administered by subcutaneous injection: 5 to 10 grams (⅛ to ⅓ ounce), according to the animal's size.

(4) For almost any kind of colic, you can give a bath or, better still, treat with a "flushing." To do this, stick the end of a garden hose into the anus and squirt in about 2 gallons of water (8 to 10 liters). This almost always works wonderfully. (See also *Bloodletting,* page 222.)

Ancient empirics used to try to cure colic by making the horse swallow a big glass of brandy into which they had crushed a well-used tobacco pipe! Actually, this isn't as far-fetched as it seems at first glance. A well-used pipe means nicotine. And nicotine increases the force and speed of intestinal motility. So if the colic is due to intestinal hypoactivity, this bizarre remedy—which was popular during the time of sorcerers—just may work.

In such a case, I recommend a somewhat updated form of this remedy. Have the horse swallow (see *How to Administer a Drug,* page 193) a decoction of a crushed package of cigarettes in a glass of brandy. In all honesty, I can't guarantee a cure.

NOTE: Before doing this, don't forget to immobilize the animal (see *Handling a horse,* page 191).

CONGESTION

A horse can have intestinal, cerebral, and—rarely—pulmonary congestion. All of these types are matters for the vet, but in an emergency, only bloodletting can save an animal stricken with cerebral congestion (see *Bloodletting,* page 222).

Pulmonary congestion

The first thing to use: mustard plasters! The surface area of a 900-pound horse requires huge amounts of powdered mustard. Take my word for it, you'll cry at least as much as you would from peeling several pounds of onions.

Then bleed the animal (see *Bloodletting,* page 222).

CONJUNCTIVITIS

This is treated as in the dog (see *Conjunctivitis,* page 77).

CONSTIPATION

Bear in mind that the horse, like all other herbivores, only defecates after light exercise; so don't assume prematurely that he's constipated.

But he may be. If so, replace his daily oats with mash (see *Injured Bars,* page 197), to which add ½ pint (about ¼ liter) of linseed—just as for a canary; only the quantity changes.

This is an excellent laxative that will set him right. If it doesn't do the job, however, an enema of soapy water or bran water may be effective. For a horse, however, you'll have to expect to use several quarts (liters).

CONTUSIONS

See *Bruises,* page 197.

HEATSTROKE

When I was a very young vet, I once went to a racetrack in Toulouse during the month of June. One of my buddies, whose parents had given him a horse, was supposed to race. He left the horse in one of those very small horse-boxes that can be attached to the back of a car, and he left him in there right up to the time when the animal had to run.

When my friend finally let him out of that torrid enclosure, you should have seen the horse's head—eyes bulging, mouth and nostrils almost black! Furthermore, he was panting, which is very unusual for a horse, and all his muscles were trembling.

Even though I was a very young vet, I didn't hesitate to diagnose this as heatstroke.

This particular case was the result of the thoughtlessness of an inexperienced horseman. It can happen sooner or later, and if you want to save the animal, don't wait for the vet but do as I did: bleed the horse (see *Bloodletting*, page 222). If the vet doesn't arrive in the meantime, you must then give a subcutaneous injection of Phenergan (promethazine hydrochloride).

The essential thing, *don't forget,* is the bloodletting.

INFECTION OF THE HOOF

This is an eczema under the nail of the horse's foot. It mainly attacks draft horses, whose stable litter leaves something to be desired. I bring it up because it is treated with copper sulfate and what I really want to tell you is this: copper sulfate is a friend of the horse's feet. It can be bought from blacksmiths. If you notice that the bottom of your horse's foot smells a little, immediately daub it with a solution of copper sulfate. This generally suffices to stop any development of eczema.

Villate liqueur (see *Rotted Fourchette*, page 212) is equally recommended.

CREVICE

This is a rope burn (see *Rope Burn,* page 221) that has been poorly taken care of. So you have to see the vet, who will treat it with antibiotic pomades.

WATER ON THE LEGS

This is when the horse—usually a draft horse—develops "thick legs."

While you wait for the vet, the only person capable of treating the animal, bathe the horse with a hot boric acid solution. (Ask the druggist for boric acid solution.)

STRAIN

". . . *Caramba!* my father said,
And the horse strained his back leg."

Well! These two famous lines prove that Victor Hugo was not a horseman and knew nothing at all about that noble beast: the horse never strains a back leg—it's impossible! He always strains his side, or else it wouldn't be a strain.

A strain is actually caused by an untoward movement: the horse dodges to avoid an obstacle and contorts himself, either in the front or the rear. It often happens to very skittish horses that are easily frightened.

Only a vet can do something about it. While you wait for him, let the horse rest and bathe the afflicted leg. (See *Kidney sores,* page 199.)

PUSTULES

This, very simply, is hives in a horse: allergic urticaria which occurs quite often in the spring. You can diagnose it very easily: the horse is all swollen and, since the condition itches him, he rubs against every available object.

Treat with injections of Phenergan (promethazine hydro-chloride). Vets have a special preparation of this medicine for horses. But if it's an emergency and injections are necessary (see *Injections*, page 220), figure a dose three times that prescribed for a person, and administer it every eight hours.

POISONING

He was a horse marked by destiny. An old nag past his prime, he pulled, with sorrowful steps and a tearful eye, one of the last hearses that wasn't motor-driven.

But he had one consolation for this lugubrious job: his master, an undertaker and bachelor like himself. They were pledged to a friendship which, although solemn, was no less profound.

The coachman always arranged for his horse to stand in the shade, after conveying the deceased to his final resting place at the cemetery.

"My horse is just as good a Christian as the deceased that is buried," declared the man. "There is no reason why he should suffer while the soul that he has just hauled is on his way to paradise." And at certain funerals, in a low voice that no one could hear, he added, "or to hell."

So in the winter he tied Mr. Horse in the sun, and during the summer, in the shade. And then he gave the signal to dig the ground.

One particular summer, he left his old companion in the shade of a large yew tree. That day the ceremony was lengthy; the deceased had gained some notoriety for himself. The horse got to thinking that the smell of the yew was kind of appetizing. In order to pass the time, he began to browse on it.

Alas! A mortal slumber followed his pangs of hunger. The yew isn't the symbol of cemeteries for nothing: it is extremely poison-ous to horses. Horses, being as foolish as people, consider it the greatest of delicacies!

So remember one thing: *never* tie a horse near a yew tree. Should this happen through someone's carelessness, call your vet at once; only he can save the animal with the aid of stimulants and laxatives. While you wait, prevent the horse from making *any* movement; this would hasten his demise.

The horse, being either more sensible or less inquisitive than the dog, doesn't go putting his nose in where it doesn't belong and so is rarely poisoned by other toxic substances.

ENTERITIS

This condition obviously is manifested by colic (see *Colic,* page 205). You can tell that it's enteritis because instead of having well-formed feces, the horse has coated feces; that is, soft and covered with a sort of mucous and transparent layer. Following this stage, the feces may become frankly liquid and resemble cow dung. Enteritis is treated as follows:

(1) Give the horse a drench of laudanum (always keep some in your veterinary medicine chest); that is, ⅓ to ½ ounce (10 to 15 grams) of laudanum in a little water.

(2) Give him an emollient to eat (see *Injured Bars* for the recipe for mash, page 197). The ancients even extolled ingesting cresol solution as an intestinal antiseptic. Laudanum, once it has relieved the pain, is generally useless.

(3) If there is no improvement, try formalin, 5 parts per thousand injected intravenously (see *Injections* for Horses, page 220).

All this is secondary to having the vet come, don't forget.

CALK

This is a farriery term that refers to the back part of a horseshoe.

It is also the veterinary medical name for a cyst along the elbow. It occurs in horses that recline with their forelegs folded in such a fashion that the leg comes in contact with the calk of the horseshoe on the same leg. (See *Hygroma of the Elbow,* page 217.) In such an event, have his farriery corrected.

ROTTED FOURCHETTE

As you may know, the fourchette is part of the horse's hoof: the frog, the part that allows him to feel the ground. An eczematous secretion can make it "rot." There are two ways to detect this:

(1) from a slight limp.
(2) from a very disagreeable odor which resembles that emitted by a dog with eczema.

Treat it by rubbing the fourchette with a medicine that your druggist can make and that, moreover, you should always keep in your veterinary medicine chest: Villate liqueur. This is its composition:

½ ounce (about 15 grams) of copper sulfate
½ ounce of zinc sulfate
1 ounce of Goulard's extract
7 ounces (about 200 grams) of white vinegar.

First dissolve the sulfates in the vinegar; then add the lead extract. Shake before using.

FRACTURE

You are aware of the horrible fate that befalls a horse that breaks a leg while racing: he is shot.

In my opinion this is barbarous. A horse that breaks a leg can be saved. He won't be able to run any more—but so what? He can still be a stud. He can also just be a contented horse in a meadow. A dog isn't obligated to be a watchdog or a retriever; he can just be a friend. Why can't we have the same attitude toward our noble companion, rather than pitilessly sending him to the slaughterhouse?

Hassan II shared my opinion on this matter. One year his favorite horse, Fackar, ran at Casablanca. A stroke of bad luck caused that handsome Anglo-Arabian to miss a turn, fall, and break his pastern.

I had come along to watch my friend Fackar, and not to act as track veterinarian. The latter, when he saw the accident, came over, examined the compound fracture, and grimaced.

"He has to be shot."

I stroked the trembling nose of the stallion, and he looked at me. He showed neither fear nor agitation, but he seemed certain of what the vet had decreed: he was going to be shot for having made that false step. I shall never forget those big blond eyes staring at me. At that instant I knew that if I let Fackar be shot, I would feel like a murderer the rest of my life.

Immediately I telephoned the king and gave him my colleague's verdict. Then the words that I was hoping to hear came over the wire:

"Out of the question! I order you to save the animal."

But there remained a problem which I had to admit to the king: no preparations for dealing with a fracture are made at a racetrack, other than providing a revolver.

"You'll manage. I have confidence in you."

I was confused—but very happy.

My horse had gotten up. He had been taken a short distance away from the racetrack and, standing on three legs, he grazed quietly, without apparent concern. The pain had, very rapidly, effectively anesthetized him.

I needed, first of all, a rubber bandage. Luckily for Fackar, I had noticed that the racetrack custodian was wearing bandages for varicose veins. I borrowed them from him—on orders of His Majesty! And with that bandage and a piece of wood that I found, I made a rude splint (see *Fracture of the Paw* in Dogs, page 61). This allowed me to get Fackar up in his horse-box and to take him to Rabat.

I had a terrific blacksmith, who had only one fault: on Sundays he got dead drunk! In the middle of the night I had to rouse him from his drunken stupor—that wasn't the easiest part of my task! With a thick tongue, he called for the "good" old method:

"To the slaughterhouse . . ."

"Listen," I said. "The king has told me to save the animal. We're going to save him!"

The words "the king" affected him like a cold shower. He emerged from his alcoholic fog and set about making what I asked of him: a piece of iron extending from under the hoof up to the knee. Once he was fully awake, he made it perfectly. Then I attached it to the horse's leg, leaving a window in front so that I could dress the wound, since it was open.

Fackar took several weeks to recover, and he lost over 300

pounds in the process. But he came out of it very well. He is still alive.

So if you ever have a horse that breaks a leg, before you shoot him think about the king's stallion—and save him.

If you have to transport him, do as I did and make a splint. The rest, obviously, is up to the vet.

Fracture of the point of the hip (dislocated hip)

The thing to do about this is to avoid it, and to do so, certain precautions should be taken.

When entering his horse-box, Horsey often clumsily dislocates his hip. He was out in bright light, he enters the shade, he can't see where to put his feet, and he runs into the door or the wall.

You should lead him into the stable at a pace that assures that he won't bump himself, rather than removing his halter and sending him in at a gallop.

MANGE

Veterinarians of old used to wait patiently while a horse of about a year old got mange and just as regularly lost it. This is now seen rarely in the horse. It is still contagious, however. Since anything can happen, here is how to treat it if your horse gets it:

(1) Shave the affected area.
(2) Rub the skin vigorously with the following mixture:
  1 pound (about 500 grams) of green soap
  ½ quart (about 500 grams) of cresol
  8 ounces (about 250 grams) of alcohol.

Repeat until healed.

STRANGLES

This is a contagious microbial disease that only affects colts. The disease usually presents itself as angina and a runny nose.

The patient should be isolated, kept in a warm spot, and given an intravenous injection of 5 parts per thousand of formalin; that is, 1.5 to 5 grams of pure formalin diluted in 20 to 50 grams (⅔ to 1¾ ounces) of distilled water.

This medicine makes the little horse so sad that he cries but the next day he is cured! These days, antibiotic therapy has replaced formalin, but if no antibiotic is available, this time-honored remedy should not be disdained.

CUTANEOUS HABRONEMIASIS

This disease only occurs in warm climates. Every summer, sores appear around the pastern. You can try to treat them in vain; they won't heal. But as soon as winter comes, they disappear. For years and years vets wondered what caused them. Then recently they found out: they are due to the larvae of a stomach worm, *Habronema,* which are transmitted by stable flies or their larvae. In the spring, the worm lays its eggs and the flies or their larvae act as intermediate hosts, transporting the worm larvae from the horse's manure to his mouth or skin, where they spend the summer maturing in comfort.

You can't treat this yourself, and even the vet will have trouble curing it. While you wait for him, content yourself with daubing the sores with methylene blue.

HEMORRHAGE

See *Wounds* in Dogs, page 95.

HERNIA

Inguinal hernia is extremely serious for the horse as a whole. The reason is that part of the intestine slips into the scrotum, which becomes visibly enlarged. Moreover, the horse has colic and is prostrated.

NOTE: This is an emergency because very soon there will be a strangulated hernia, and then . . . no more horse. But this is a matter solely for the vet, because the animal must be castrated.

HYGROMA OF THE ELBOW

This is a cyst which forms subsequent to a callosity usually due to constant repetition of a movement. Thus devout nuns have hygroma of the knee, and tailors used to get it on the medial surface of the lower leg.

The horse gets them when, thinking he's a cow, he lies down like one. Actually, our noble beast isn't supposed to lie down at all; he's even supposed to sleep standing up. However, if he does allow himself to stretch out, it will be on his flank. Now some of them, perversely, lie down on their legs, as you have often seen cows do in meadows. This is certainly degrading for the equine race, but it is also very serious because it can give rise to callosities which rapidly become enormous cysts that bother the horse when he moves.

He then must be taken to the vet, who will have plenty of difficulty curing him.

So what you should do isn't to treat hygroma but avoid it. To do so, provide a horse that is lying down in this fashion with very thick stable litter so that his legs will be padded by straw, which will prevent formation of these cysts.

INDIGESTION

See *Colic,* page 205.

SKIN IRRITATION

This is often observed following shaving. Unlike a dog, a domestic horse must be shaved, in the winter.

This may seem peculiar at first, but it is easily explained. The horse, like all animals, grows a thicker coat for winter which is warmer than his summer one. With the advent of civilization, he now lives in a warm stable. But, unlike carnivores that in a comparable situation lose their fur, he keeps his.

The result: if you don't shave a horse that is too warm, he sweats—which doesn't happen to felines or canids—and the sweat accumulates on the skin and hair, leading to chills and congestion.

He must be shaved in the winter to avoid this.

However, it happens that shaving causes a kind of hives in the animal. He then must be rubbed down with medicinal boric acid. This usually does the job.

INJURIES

For all injuries, whether bruises, tendinitis, cannon sores, boulet, or whatever, you should *cool warm wounds and heat cool wounds.*

While you await the vet this is the only thing to do, but it is absolutely necessary that you do it!

If you are an accomplished horseman, I assume that you know how to recognize a warm or a cool wound: by feeling the area that seems to be affected, with the back of your hand.

To *heat* a wound, use hot poultices of linseed or mustard.

To *cool* a wound, there is only one way: to hose the horse down with a garden hose until you can't hold it up any longer.

In the case of leg injuries, another very good thing to do—if you live near the sea—is to walk your horse along the water's edge.

RIB INJURY

This is due to a kick in the ribs that a horse receives from a buddy who is in a bad mood; it results in a fracture. (See *Fracture,* page 213.)

It is then absolutely essential to prevent the horse from breathing normally; otherwise, healing is impeded.

To do so, rub him down with a vesicatory ointment in the area of the fracture (all blacksmiths have this). Since it is extremely painful stuff, especially during inspiration or expiration, the horse, in order to minimize his discomfort, will alter his respiratory movements and breathe through his abdomen. Thus the ribs are immobilized. Moreover, the influx of blood stimulated by the blistering agent also enhances healing of the fracture.

OVERREACH CUT OR TENDINITIS

This is a strained tendon. It occurs either following a kick from another horse or following exertion, as when the animal has run too much. You will be able to detect it when the horse returns to the stable. A horseman's trained eye will observe that the back of the tendon is "pot-bellied." Old veterinarians referred to it as "trout stomach."

Like splints, these are matters for the vet, but while you are waiting for him, suppress the inflammation in the way described for injuries (see *Injuries*, page 218).

OPHTHALMIA

If the horse's eye tears or is red, wash it with the following lotion:

1 pint (about 500 grams) of marshmallow decoction
2 grams of alum
2 grams of camphorated brandy.

In cases of chronic ophthalmia, have the following solution prepared by the druggist:

1 ounce (about 32 grams) of slaked lime
4 grams of powdered ammonium chloride
1 gram of cinnamon powder
2 grams of Armenian bole powder
1 gram of powdered cloves
1 gram of powdered vegetable charcoal.

This isn't an eye salve but a powder that you blow on the eyes.

If your horse has a foreign object in his eye—dust or a gnat— rub the following decoction in the eye; it's a good, astringent eye salve

2 handfuls of plantain leaves
½ handful of young bramble-bush thorns
15 grams of crushed oak bark
4 grams of table salt
1 quart (liter) of water.

INJECTIONS

A horse is usually only given a subcutaneous injection for an artificial abscess.

Intramuscular injections: These are made in the flat surface of the neck and are the kind most frequently employed because they are very easy to administer. There is, in fact, a little trick that you can use so that the horse doesn't feel anything. Lead him out by the halter; that's all you need. Then pet him, giving him some good smacks on the neck—he loves that. Then, between slaps, quickly stick in the needle. He won't notice a thing.

Horsemen sometimes object to this technique, claiming that such injections may diminish the suppleness of the delicate balance that the neck constitutes. So if the injections are, for example, too numerous or too irritating, give them in the rump: in the "right upper quadrant" so dear to nurses. But *beware!* Stand off to the side if you don't want a rare but ultimately inevitable kick to knock you over.

Intravenous injections: It is actually possible to give a horse an intravenous injection. They are always given in the jugular; you proceed as you do for bloodletting, making sure, obviously, that the horse can't budge.

(1) Make the jugular stand out by pushing on it with the flat of your hand. If this doesn't work sufficiently, loop a rope around the horse's neck and tighten it so that the vein stands out.

(2) The jugular is very large and obvious, so you won't have any trouble sticking in the needle and making the injection.

NOTE: It's advisable to use very large needles when giving injections to horses.

OPEN WOUNDS

It can never be overemphasized: an open wound in a horse should release an immediate reflex in the horseman: tetanus antitoxin! Of all animals, the horse is the most likely to have this awful disease, which will unfailingly kill him if he isn't given an injection in time. It shouldn't be forgotten that the tetanus bacillus lives best in horse manure.

Tetanus antitoxin works perfectly well *preventatively* in the horse.

The vet, of course, is much more likely than you to be treating the wound, but it's up to you not to take it lightly, expecting that it won't amount to anything. (See also *Tetanus,* page 226.)

ROPE BURN

The horse's ear itched. He scratched it with his back foot—and clumsily caught it in the tether to which he was tied! He got alarmed, pulled back, and of course injured his pastern.

His owner, fortunately, noticed it and cleaned the small wound with a 10% solution of cresol; that did the trick. But if he hadn't seen it in time, a crevice would have formed, and that would have been much more troublesome. (See *Crevice,* page 210.)

PRURITIS OF THE ANAL REGION

I recall an amusing spectacle: riding astride the stud one morning, I saw a young colt with his tail all mussed up. It made him look rather ridiculous but at the same time endearing, like a horse in an animated cartoon.

Anyway, thanks to that plume I knew right away what was wrong: he had anal pruritis, which itched him so during the night that in order to scratch it he rubbed against the wall—which gave him that frizzy tail.

Pruritis under the tail has several possible causes:

(1) The horse has been badly groomed and his harness has hurt him.

(2) It may be due to the presence of botfly larvae.

(3) Ascaris.

In the case of (1), the horse has to be left without his harness until he is healed, and then you have to make sure that it doesn't hurt him again.

In the case of (2) or (3), the parasites must be killed. To do so, follow the old remedy of making the horse take 2 grams of arsenic a day.

It is difficult to obtain this potent poison today; formerly it was sold as easily as baking soda. If you aren't able to get some without having the FBI after you, give the horse ½ to 2 ounces (about 15 to 60 grams) of oil of turpentine in a drinkable solution every day (see *How To Administer a Drug*, page 193).

Since there is no emergency, ask your vet for an antihelmintic. Nowadays there are some very powerful ones that are perfectly innocuous.

BLOODLETTING

Bleeding is something of the universal panacea of the physicians of Molière.

As with humans in the seventeenth century, bleeding was formerly done for horses against every disease, from inflammation of the foot to congestion.

But if man has renounced this treatment for himself, he hasn't given it up for his companion. The horse should be bled—not for every condition under the sun, but in very serious cases it can save his life: congestion, of course, but also infections (reasonably enough, if you withdraw 3 to 5 quarts of blood from the horse, you remove a proportional amount of the toxin).

It is best to leave this procedure to the vet, but in an emergency—heatstroke for example (see *Heatstroke*, page 209)—you should know how to perform it.

To do so, you need a special trocar for bloodletting. Carry one in your veterinary medicine chest (see *Medicine Chest for a*

Horse, page 230). It consists of a very large needle that is beveled on three sides, which slides inside a metal tube. Now here is what to do:

(1) Hold the horse (see *Handling a horse,* page 191).

(2) With the flat of your hand, push upward to make the jugular stand out (this is the large vein on each side of the neck); you can feel it very easily under your hand. If you don't succeed, slip a rope around the horse's breast and tighten it to the extent necessary.

(3) Take the trocar and plunge the whole thing, sheath and all, into the jugular. Withdraw the needle by pulling on the handle which is found at the end of the shaft of the needle. The little steel tube which remains embedded in the vein will thus allow the blood to flow out.

(4) Withdraw from 3 to 5 quarts (liters) of blood, according to the animal's size and physical state. The latter is determined, in cases of congestion, from the appearance of the animal's eyes: when the horse needs to be bled, the whites of the eyes are congested. You withdraw just enough blood for the eyes to become normal.

(5) When enough blood has been withdrawn, remove the tube from the jugular.

(6) Since this makes a good-sized hole, it may not close. If it doesn't, push the edges of the hole together and fasten them closed with a strong safety pin, which will work as an agraffe.

It may happen—in a case of heatstroke, for example—that you have no trocar available. If you don't:

(1) Make the jugular stand out with a rope.

(2) With a razor blade make an incision in the vein about 2 inches (5 centimeters) long.

(3) The blood will gush out. Withdraw about 3 to 5 quarts and then close the wound.

(4) To do this, take some very large safety pins and close it up, impaling not only the skin but also the wall of the vein.

It should be obvious that this type of operation should only be performed in an emergency. The horse loses a great deal of his blood; don't you lose *your* sangfroid!

NOTE: Only bleed a horse that can stand it. If he is weak, undernourished, or in poor health, you must not do it because it will exhaust him.

I remind you that the weight of a normal horse is from about 900 to 1100 pounds (400 to 500 kilograms).

LEECHES

If you live in a warm country or climate, there may be leeches in the streams.

I became acquainted with them in Algeria where I did my military service, like a spahi. I crossed a wadi on my horse and, coming out of the water, saw that the poor beast had become the living prey of these little vampires. He had them on all the most sensitive spots: the cheeks, the soft palate, the nostrils. . . . I later learned that mares even get them in the vagina!

My horse was beside himself, and I was no less upset. As soon as I returned to camp, I got them off by hosing the places where they were attached, using saltwater. This is the only way to get rid of them!

These same leeches were employed by vets in former times in an interesting way. They immersed run-down horses in a "leech pond" half way up the cannon, thus administering a medicinal localized blood-letting, which appeared to be efficacious.

WIRE-HEEL

Wire-heel is a constant sore of the surface of the hoof. It is due to the fact that the hoof hasn't been adequately greased (especially in dry regions), so that the nail cracks.

The horse's hooves should, in fact, be greased every day. Ask the horsemen of Saumur; it's their first job of the day and if, at inspection, the hooves of the lead horses don't shine, they really catch it!

Some special ointments are sold, but you can make one yourself in the following manner:

Mix:

4½ pounds (about 2 kilograms) of horse fat
4 ounces (about 500 grams) of wax
2 pounds (about 1 kilogram) of white resin (sold by druggists).

There is nothing special about white resin; it's merely very thick, undiluted turpentine.

Melt over a low flame and then apply.

You can also use the following ancient but nevertheless excellent ointment:

2 parts yellow wax
3 parts liquid pitch
12 parts lamb tallow or lard (pork fat).

Spread on the hoof daily.

SPLINT OF THE CANNON

The horse's cannon bone is the equivalent of the metatarsal or metacarpal of man, an extremely fragile bone. From time to time a horse will kick his neighbor in the cannon. You can't take care of it, of course, but there is one thing that you can and should do: as soon as you notice the slightest deformity of the cannon, take your horse to the vet immediately, before it becomes too serious!

THRUSH

Contrary to what you may believe, this is a modern-day ailment. It occurred much less frequently in early days, when horsemen would wash their animals' grooming equipment and trappings assiduously. Nowadays, people are prone to forget these basic sanitary practices; they take one horse's saddle and put it on another, and *voilà*—thrush appears once again!

You may know that this is a fungus that multiplies rapidly and always in the form of a circle. This produces round, white patches which enlarge from the center outwards, just like a mushroom bed! The horse's hair falls out, and frequently scabs are formed.

Thrush must be treated as soon as it appears. Highly effective preparations now exist, but you can still use this old remedy:

(1) Wash the patches with a 1/1000 solution of cresol.
(2) Then rub on a 1/1000 solution of corrosive sublimate. You can find it at any drugstore.

NOTE:

(a) Thrush, slightly contagious for man, is very contagious for the horse. Therefore everything that the horse has had a chance to touch, as well as the area where he lives, must be disinfected.
(b) Never use water to treat or to wash the horse. Humidity makes fungi thrive.

TEMPERATURE

Contrary to what you probably assume, draft horses have a higher body temperature than saddle horses, even though the latter are the more high-strung. Those are the facts; no explanation is known for them.

Draft horse: 100.4°F (38°C) and above.

Saddle horse: around 99.3°F (37.4°C).

It should be noted that English thoroughbreds—those extraordinary racing horses—have the lowest temperature of saddle horses.

This means that a "horse's fever" isn't just an idle expression: when he is sick, the horse's temperature easily reaches 104°F (40°C)! You can tell he is sick by taking his temperature, just as you would for a dog or a human. So that you won't get kicked, take the precautions suggested under *Handling a horse,* page 191.

TETANUS

This is the worst of diseases for the horse. You may be aware that the bacteria of tetanus develop best and fastest in horse manure, so of course he is their foremost victim.

It is *absolutely* necessary to have a horse vaccinated every year, for—make no mistake about it—a horse stricken by tetanus is a dead horse. No treatment can save him.

I advise you further that if you borrow a horse and he sustains a wound, albeit benign, immediately give him some preventative serum; his owner may have forgotten to have him vaccinated.

TORTICOLLIS

The big bay horse took off badly on his jump: instead of leaping, he fell. Having not done himself any harm and being a little annoyed, he got up at once.

However, when he got up on his feet, it was in vain that he tried to hold his head straight: it listed to the left. He looked at me with a worried expression: what had happened to him? To reassure him I patted his neck:

"You have torticollis, old boy. Don't worry, we'll fix it and in 48 hours it will be all gone."

In getting up, he had jammed a cervical vertebra, giving him wryneck.

A horse's neck is extremely powerful and it aids his every movement; it is truly his "balance." When he falls and tries to get up, his neck bears the force that allows him to regain his feet. But in extending this effort, his neck sustains torticollis quite easily. The result: he holds his head to one side.

In a case like this, do what I did to my horse that day:

(1) Hold the head in a good position. To do so, tie one end of a sturdy elastic rope to the halter and the other to the saddle girth so that the head is gradually straightened out—but allow *some* freedom of movement.

(2) Massage the neck with an ointment or lotion.

(3) Apply a hot linseed poultice; this will help relax the muscles.

(4) Let the horse rest in a warm place while you continue the treatment, three or four times a day, until everything is back to normal.

TRACHEOTOMY

This is up to the vet, but in an emergency you can perform it just as you would for a dog (see *Tracheotomy*, page 106). Use a larger trocar, of course.

The trocar should be left in the trachea so that the horse can breathe. Nevertheless, the vet has to come right away, for the horse will have great difficulty breathing through such a small hole.

THE GRIPES

This is very violent colic. The horse's breathing is rapid and audible, and is accompanied by muscular tremors: his body is reacting with signs of anxiety. At last, overcome by pain, the horse throws himself to the ground.

The best treatment is bleeding (see *Bloodletting*, page 222).

Formalin, 5 parts per thousand, injected into the vein, has also been used successfully (see also *Colic*, page 205).

ULCERATION OF THE CORNEA

I was serving as the veterinarian of the king of Morocco when there was an epidemic of corneal ulcers among his horses.

Believe me, you get a funny feeling when a horse turns his beautiful blond eye toward you and you notice that, beside the pupil, there is a hole in the cornea. When a second and then a third horse have the same surprise in store for you, you get chills down your spine.

I imagine that the epidemic was due to the blooming of the fig trees of Barbary. Airborne pollen is apt to irritate a horse's eye and cause an ulcer.

I had ordered all sorts of miracle pomades from France and had my assistant apply them religiously three times a day, but nothing came of it and I began to get really annoyed.

A blacksmith at the stables followed my efforts with such a

mocking attitude that after a month of getting nowhere and being just about driven to distraction, I asked him:

"All right, wise guy, what would you do in my place, eh?"

"Oh," he replied calmly, "when that happens to one of my horses, I treat it with sugar."

He had a wry little smile on his face.

"Of course, I'm not a veterinarian. Naturally, you can save them much better than I. . . ."

After entertaining himself at my expense, the good fellow explained his procedure to me. He took a quarter of a lump of sugar and crushed it up as fine as he could, until the sugar approached the texture of face powder. Then he put it in a little paper funnel which he held near the horse's eye—and he blew!

It was best if no one stood in back of the horse, because the animal reared back drolly when he got the stuff in the eye!

The procedure was repeated daily.

Well, the results were extraordinary: five days later my horses were cured.

NOTE: This does not interfere with pharmaceutical treatment; it multiplies its effectiveness by a factor of 10.

Subsequently I treated corneal ulcers in dogs this way and obtained results that were just as astonishing.

I believe that the sugar attracts white blood cells to the region of the cornea, thus aiding the immune reaction. That is the only medical explanation that I can think of, but whatever the mechanism, the fact is that it does work.

WINDGALL

This is the name for an inflammation around a synovial joint.

First type: To decrease the friction where the two bones of the foot meet at the fetlock joint, between them is a little sac filled with a liquid called synovial fluid (as man has).

If the horse has exerted himself, there is an overflow of synovial fluid. This is articular windgall and it is very serious.

Second type: There are also little synovial sacs along the tendons; the fluid escapes somehow and lubricates the tendons. If the overflow of synovial fluid occurs here, the condition is called tendinous windgall, and it's nothing to be too concerned about.

Both types can be diagnosed from the bumps that appear; their size reflects how long the horse has had windgall. You should immediately:

(1) Let the horse rest.
(2) Hose down his feet (see *Kidney sores*, page 199).
(3) Call the vet.

MEDICINE CHEST FOR A HORSE

ammonia
carbolic acid
emetic (ask a vet)
laudanum
sulfuric ether
camphorated brandy
Goulard's extract
paregoric elixir
Villate liqueur
cresol
copper sulfate solution
boric acid
linseed
powdered mustard
tincture of iodine
foot ointment (see *Wire-heel*, page 224)
ophthalmic ointment (see *Ophthalmia*, page 219)
trocar for bleeding
syringe: at least 20 cubic centimeters
needles: 1½ millimeters in diameter
and most important: tetanus antitoxin (several ampoules in
    reserve)
gag and enema for administering drugs
gear for *Handling a horse,* page 191.

▸ BIRDS

An artist could gather together all the birds and paint a canvas, using only their feathers for pigment.

Struck by the songs that they sing—each one different according to the species—the musician Olivier Messiaen wrote one of his most beautiful symphonies.

Birds can be tiny, the size of a nut, like the hummingbird. They can be immense, with a wingspread attaining almost seven yards, like the condor, giant eagle of the Andes. They may feed on a spot of dew or on a cadaver—yet they are brothers.

They obey certain rules which mystify man and yet which bear a resemblance to his own laws. One day I saw a flock of crows fly overhead for twenty minutes. They were grouped in uniform squadrons, each led by a chief. Other black birds flew in position on either side, bumping aside any who seemed to want to goof off. Farther back came the slowpokes, the nonconformists, and the weaklings. The airborne traffic cops remaining among them would attack them with beaks and wings, cawing insults all the while, and would restore order to the group of stragglers, forcing them to take the proper route and flying behind and beside them in order to keep them in line.

They can communicate with each other admirably. One winter in an Irish village, an extraordinary event took place.

At dawn, the milkman left a bottle of milk sealed with an aluminum cap in front of each house. One of the villagers noticed that his bottle wasn't completely full and that the cap was torn open, so he registered a complaint. The milkman swore that he wasn't responsible for the occurrence.

Several days later a second bottle was attacked, and then a third, and then a fourth. Before a month had passed, all the bottles were being broken open and their levels of milk lowered.

The village, which wasn't Irish for nothing, began to whisper about ghosts. They lay in wait in vain; they saw nothing. The milkman delivered his milk at 6 o'clock. At 6:30 when the first shutters opened, the bottles had mysteriously been attacked.

Lying in wait behind their windows, the villagers decided to all stand guard one night.

And they saw—not a pale vampire flying out of the cemetery, but a bird that landed on the bottle, tore open the cap with a practiced stroke of its beak, drank as much as he could, and then flew off. The whole thing only lasted a few seconds.

All of the quarts of milk were visited in this manner by birds who went straight to "their" bottle.

This is what must have happened. At the beginning, a single bird one day, no doubt out of curiosity, had torn open the aluminum and, tasting the liquid, found that he liked it. So he had done it again; nothing surprising so far.

But he must then have advertised this to the other birds, leading them to the village early in the morning so that he could show them how to open a bottle. That was the enigma.

The behavior of our "fine feathered friends" is as endearing as it is astonishing. That is why a bird lover who starts off with a simple canary very often winds up, after a while, with a whole aviary.

HOW TO BUY A BIRD

Unfortunately, some bird sellers are no better than some dog merchants.

This is particularly true for parrots. They order their "merchandise" from Africa or South America in bulk amounts, without concerning themselves with "attrition"—the birds that die en route—knowing that, at the going price of a Gabon or an Amazon, they will recoup their losses with those that survive—even if the birds' subsequent survival is uncertain!

The wild parrots are caught in the forests by natives with immense nets. Then they are packed in boxes and sped to Europe.

It is obvious that a bird so traumatized will often be victimized by a disease—usually pulmonary congestion—or by stress. The customer has bought a nice, gentle bird; he doesn't know that the parrot is like that only because he is sick. If he is healthy, it takes a good month before he gets used to his human family. And until he is tamed, you have to be wary of his pecking!

Don't believe that a parrot seeking shelter in the hollow of your hand without knowing you is "gentle" or "adorable"; he is simply sick.

This is particularly true for captured wild birds. Canaries, goldfinches, cut-throat weavers, etc. that have been raised in cages and have reproduced in them for generations are almost always in good shape.

Lastly—and very fortunately—it isn't necessary to put all bird sellers in the same cage. Some are very conscientious and love their work; you will find their birds to be in excellent health.

So, as with dogs and cats, you have to know how to select a bird when you shop. Never take a bird:

whose droppings are liquid (except for frugivores, principally the toucan)
whose feathers are ruffled
whose respiration is labored
whose eyes are half-closed
that is rolled up in a ball.

Purchase a bird whose cheerful appearance and vivacity indicate that he is in good health.

HANDLING

How to catch and hold a bird to treat it

When I was a young man, my fencing instructor used to tell me: "Hold the foil like a bird: if you hold it too tightly it suffocates; if you hold it too loosely it flies away."

Later, when I became a vet and had to hold birds, I understood better still what he had meant.

First, when you have to treat a bird:

(1) catch him;

(2) keep him in your hands without suffocating him but without letting him fly away. Before anything else, you have to learn how to take hold of him. To do so:

(a) Close all the windows and doors, because if he gets away from you. . . .

(b) Get rid of everything on which he could perch beyond your reach: curtain rods, etc. If you don't, you can spend all day chasing him.

(c) If your bird is in his cage, stick your hand inside and gently but firmly grasp the bird and gather him in. You must hold his wings; if not, one may break. Leave only the two feet and the head free.

NOTE: If you have an aviary, it is best to first use a butterfly net to catch him; then grasp him as I have just indicated. This is the procedure for small birds like canaries. Never grab a bird by the end of the wing; at best you will have a bird without feathers on one side, at worst one with a broken wing.

If you have to deal with a biting parakeet, hold his neck between your index and middle fingers. This will allow him to turn his head but not to pinch you with his beak. The maneuver will be very handy for you in *Sharpening the Beak* (see page 264).

These same parakeets also get foot mange. To treat them, push them into a cardboard tube from which only the head and feet stick out; you will then be able to care for the latter easily. Use the same procedure to cut a bird's nails.

For very large birds—macaws, cockatoos, Great Amazons—it is best to have leather gloves (fowler gloves or, instead, soldering gloves). For even if they are very tame and like their owner, they will rebel if he tries to meddle in some matter which, in their opinion, doesn't concern him.

Large parrots are very strong, so they have to be held securely. To do so, two people are needed. Your helper grasps the bird the way you hold hens out in the country: after placing its body under his left arm and pressing it between his arm and his side, he takes its neck in his right hand. The bird is thus totally immobilized—which, I warn you, puts him in a very bad humor. But this is the only way that he can be cared for.

In order to administer a pill, which is quite often necessary, you also need two people. While one person holds the bird in the manner I have just described, the other teases its beak with the handle of a spoon. Already furious, the parrot at once takes out his anger by seizing the handle. All that remains is to turn the handle so it is vertical. The bird finds itself with its beak wedged open and all you have to do is to slip the pill into the corner of its beak; the bird will be forced to swallow it.

If by chance you find a diurnal or nocturnal bird of prey that is injured and you want to save it, you will have to grab it as you would a parrot. But be even more careful: its talons are more formidable than the powerful claws of a cockatoo! Remember that it is with these that it catches its prey. An eagle is capable of lifting up and carrying off a lamb.

However, there is a very simple way to handle screech owls, and you can also use it on turtledoves even though they are a very different bird. Turn the bird over on its back and it won't budge. This explains in part how magicians perform their tricks.

Small birds: this includes birds ranging from the canary to the parrot and including the cuckoo, widow bird, etc.

The pathology of all these birds is identical, so I won't give you any special remedies for the canary or for the robin. They are all cared for in the same way.

THE SICK BIRD

It is very difficult, especially when you're inexperienced, to detect illness of any kind in a bird. Birds don't exhibit their suffering the way mammals do, nor do they complain by wailing like a dog or a cat. So you have to rely on their general appearance to tell you that something is wrong.

(1) They roll up into a ball in a corner and don't budge. Their feathers are ruffled and they themselves are sad and crestfallen.

(2) If the bird has a cold or a pulmonary ailment, his beak will be agape so he can breathe.

(3) If there is a digestive problem the droppings are liquid. However, frugivorous birds such as toucans, lories, and grackles always have liquid droppings.

(4) The nostrils are often purulent, and the eyes glaucous or shut.

It is useless to take the bird's temperature, even if it's a large bird that would be able to accept the thermometer: the normal temperature is between 105.8 and 111.2°F (41 to 44°C).

Treatment should be begun as soon as the first of these symptoms appears. This is especially true if the bird is small, since his size renders him more delicate.

If the bird has been kept with other birds, it must immediately be isolated because the disease may be contagious.

ACARIASIS

This is caused by a small parasite, a tick that inhabits the trachea and bronchi of the bird. As contented as a sheep in green pastures, it "grazes" on the trachea, causing chattering of the bird's beak and difficult respiration accompanied by coughing and sneezing.

All small birds without exception can be victims of this tick. This is a recent disease only described in 1948, and only a vet is able to treat it.

BROKEN WING

This is an absolutely incredible animal story, told to me by one of my clients, Mrs. G. Although it has a rather sad ending, at least it is quite uplifting.

"It was a blue and white spring afternoon. I was crossing the Luxembourg Gardens when I heard some little cries. On the grass a young blackbird was cheeping as loudly as she could and dragging her wing. Doubtless she had broken it by flying out of her nest when she was still unsteady on her wings.

"I extended my hand. She let herself be picked up as though she sensed that my hand was that of a savior."

Thus Blackbird was taken home by Mrs. G. Fortunately, the

young bird already knew how to feed itself; this spared my client the totally absorbing attention that an unweaned bird demands (see *Bird Fallen from a Nest,* page 251). Another problem existed: Mrs. G. already had a dog and a cat. The young woman decided to put her whole menagerie together, under observation to be sure, in order to see what would happen. The results were satisfactory. The dog turned right on his heel, shrugging his shoulders. He had already seen everything in that crazy house, from a guinea pig to a tame snake! As for the cat, this was a Burmese who became nursemaid to a canary, as I shall describe further on (see *Broken Leg,* page 254). He obviously found the bird bigger than a canary but friendly, since he was purring softly.

Reassured, Mrs. G. bandaged the blackbird's wing and placed her under the cat's medical observation. Everything went very well until the day when the bird was healed. Her guardian took her to the Luxembourg Gardens in order to set her free, but the blackbird would have nothing to do with the plan, returning immediately to the young woman's hands.

"I had no idea that a bird could perspire," she exclaimed to me, "but she was dripping with sweat, just like someone seized by panic!"

So Blackbird was returned to Mrs. G.'s house where she resumed her happy life with her four-legged friends.

The cat was her real pal. She was always with him, her favorite pastime consisting of perching on his head. Thus crowned, the Burmese—retaining his dignity and never forgetting that he was a sacred cat—continued to go about his business. When you got close to him, you could hear him purring.

One morning, this entire charming menagerie left for the country in order to spend the summer there. Even though she had a garden at her disposal, Blackbird never thought of fleeing.

Sometimes she would perch on a branch so as to tease the cat by jumping down on him when he passed below.

Then one morning she couldn't be found. Everyone searched, called. It was the Burmese that discovered what remained of his friend: a foot and several feathers. Not being suspicious of cats, the bird had allowed one of the neighborhood cats to approach her, and he had "loved" her after his fashion.

"The Burmese didn't eat for two days. Overcome by sorrow, he hid under a bush and didn't even go into the house. He was also lying in wait: we understood this when we were awakened at dawn by the screeching of a cat fight."

Patiently, the Burmese had awaited his enemy who, thinking that perhaps there was another blackbird to eat, had returned to the scene of the crime. But this time the scoundrel received the most punishing drubbing that a cat ever got. The Burmese left him almost dead and then, satisfied, returned home, ate something, and resumed his life.

If you ever either have or find a bird whose wing is broken, here is how you should proceed to repair it:

(1) Pick up the bird very gently so as not to exacerbate the damage, grasping the side that isn't hurt.

(2) If the fracture is open as is often the case, the wound is generally *under* the wing. It must be disinfected with hydrogen peroxide.

(3) The important thing is to prevent the bird from flying. To do so, you have to tie the wing rather tightly against his body by means of gauze or even a little adhesive band-aid that you can later remove with ether. But don't tighten it too much or you will suffocate the bird.

(4) Isolate him by putting him in a box for at least ten days.

(5) When the wing has healed, remove the bandage and set him free or return him to his aviary.

Certain wing fractures cannot be treated in this manner; for example, those in which the ends of the bone are too far out of line. In these cases veterinary surgery is called for. Prosthetic bones for birds are now manufactured!

ASPERGILLOSIS

Even though this disease is solely a matter for the vet, I mention it because in its initial stages it can be easily confused with bronchitis.

The diseased bird dies between three and five days, so this is an emergency. The pheasant and raptorial birds are among the species most easily stricken.

Lastly and especially if you have a bird that wakes up with aspergillosis, since this disease is contagious, immediately wash and disinfect his cage or aviary, making very sure that you don't leave any food debris. The disease is actually due to mildew that invades the respiratory tract, and food particles allow mildew to develop.

ASTHMA

Rarely does a small bird get this, and if he does have it he will die before you even have time to detect it. It isn't the same for large birds.

BULIMIA

The bird eats and then eats some more, then he wastes away and finally dies.

You think that it's a psychosomatic disease—and it is, just like in a human being.

There can be two mutually exclusive explanations for this.

Either the bird is bored or lives in an aviary that has too many inhabitants! Whatever the cause, it's a disease of teals.

If it's an aviary bird, it must be separated immediately from the others, because the disease is contagious.

Moreover, all psychiatrists know that a suicide on the immediate premises often leads to others.

In both types of bulimia, it is necessary to:

(1) Put the little animal's cage out in the sunlight.

(2) Change its food—rusk in milk and egg yolk is excellent—and sprinkle its seed with a pinch of kitchen salt.

(3) Distract it. Spend time with it; put on classical music records: songbirds love music.

(4) Show the bird to the vet at your earliest opportunity. He will prescribe amino acids, which are indispensable in these cases.

CONSTIPATION

You can tell a bird is constipated when:

(1) Its droppings are very hard and dry, rather than being slightly soft.

(2) The number of droppings decreases. Thus the parakeet excretes a minimum of 30; anything below this figure signifies constipation.

(3) The tail feathers surrounding the cloaca are dry.

(4) The bird's belly is swollen.

The constipation may be due simply to eating. In the parakeet it is often due to egg mash, of which it is very fond and which it eats in excessive amounts.

In the other birds, usually hempseed is responsible. That is why, rather than preparing your birds' menu yourself, it is better to buy it at a pet shop. There are people who specialize in feeding birds; they know just what seeds suit each species.

Treat constipation as follows:

For small, granivorous birds: Put a piece of sulfur in their water. Mix rapeseed, poppyseed, and lettuce seed in their food. Give them some green vegetables; lettuce is excellent as long as you don't give too much and run the risk of producing an effect opposite to that desired.

Combat the constipation quickly, or else the bird's exertions may lead to *Inversion of the Cloaca* (see page 256).

For the parakeet: Add fruit and green vegetables to the diet. Give it three drops of paraffin oil with each meal.

Don't forget that avian pathology is very special. Become familiar with your birds; don't merely observe them from a distance. This will allow you to detect the first sign of trouble and to modify their diet in one way or another.

COMMON COLD

The writer Louis-Ferdinand Céline loved animals. In his house he reserved the ground floor for dogs, the second floor for cats; as for the birds, they had to be satisfied with the more modest quarters of the bathroom.

I often went to see him because that menagerie demanded constant care, and each time he said to me inconsolably:

"Two more canaries are dead. It was bound to happen: I kept telling the maid not to let in any drafts but she didn't listen to me, so of course the birds caught cold!"

Coryza is fatal to small birds. A draft of air and no more canary! It is much more important to prevent the disease than to try to cure it—which is almost impossible because there isn't sufficient time to do so.

Even when they do take precautions, people don't do so sufficiently. The cage is placed in front of an open window, or a door is opened, and there is a 50:50 chance that the ensuing breeze will spell the end of the little bird.

Ice water should not be put in the birdbath. In winter, if the tap water is cold, add hot water so that it is at least at room temperature.

Be suspicious of your guests. The friend who takes the ice cube out of his drink and, not knowing where to deposit it, puts it in the bird's trough is a murderer.

Nevertheless, there is a way of treating your canary before the cold manifests itself, if you think the bird has caught a chill. My colleague Dr. Philippe de Wailly, a bird specialist, came up with the idea: add 2 drops of whiskey to 10 drops of water and give it to the bird to drink.

I recall that when I was a boy my mother, when she saw that our cut-throat weaver which we had then looked peaked, put a little red wine on a lump of sugar which she placed in the cage. Our feathered drunkard loved it, and I always suspected that the bird pretended to be sick in order to get it. In any case, the treatment was very successful.

Try whiskey or red wine, depending on your bird's taste. If the bird isn't willing to take it straight (generally they love sugar soaked in wine), catch it (see 233) and give the medicine either with the aid of an eyedropper that you stick into the side of its beak or with a wad of cotton soaked with the liquid, rolled onto the end of a little stick, and introduced into the beak. The bird bites down in order to get rid of the stick, squeezes the cotton, and swallows the liquid.

Needless to say, the bird should be put in a warm place (77 to 86°F or 25 to 30°C) where there is no draft.

DIARRHEA

If you notice that a bird has liquid droppings, separate it from the others, as I have already said, for this can imply an infectious or parasitic disease.

It can, of course, be less serious; the bird may have eaten too much roughage, or may merely have gotten chilled or have drunk something cold, as with coryza (see *Common Cold,* page 240).

Treatment of diarrhea is very simple:

(1) Add 3 or 4 drops of paregoric elixer to the bird's drinking water. Put the same amount in the birdbath because it often drinks just as much from there as from the trough. If the bird is quite large—a turtledove or parrot, etc.—introduce 4 drops of elixer directly into the beak.

(2) Sprinkle a good-sized pinch of powdered bismuth subnitrate onto his food for several days.

If these steps don't bring quick improvement, you'll have to see the vet because it may be:

(1) *Coccidiosis:* a serious and contagious parasitic disease which the vet alone can treat. It is characterized by reddish diarrhea.

(2) *Salmonellosis:* the classic green diarrhea of birds. As contagious as coccidiosis, this disease is microbial.

HOARSENESS IN SONGBIRDS

If you have several songbirds in a cage or in the same aviary, it is very possible that one morning you will notice that one of your birds is sounding an appalling false note instead of delighting your ears with its warbling.

It is hoarse.

This is nothing to be worried about. Being as vain as operatic tenors, avian vocalists try to prove their voices superior to all others. So they trill, warble, and otherwise emit their shrillest notes, seeking incessantly to dominate their rivals. As a result, they become hoarse.

Set such a bird apart from the others and put a teaspoonful of honey in its water. After several days it will have recovered its voice and you will be able to put it back with the others—until the next time!

MANGE

Parakeet foot mange

The blue parakeet's feet had doubled in size. She scratched them with her beak until they bled. She had mange!

This still occurs quite frequently. The bird should be treated with an oily solution obtainable at pet shops or, failing that, at the vet's.

Beak mange

If you don't treat foot mange in time, it will be transmitted to the bird's beak. This is fatal because the bird scratches itself with its beak, and before long the mange gets into its eyes. Obviously, there is only one solution: treat the feet and beak at the same time. But I implore you not to leave Madame Parakeet in this state: she suffers greatly!

Body mange

This, fortunately, is a very rare disease. At the beginning you may mistake it for the onset of moulting since it makes the bird's feathers fall out—except that only the small feathers of the wings and of the tail come loose. This detail is what gives it away. But I repeat, this condition is quite unusual. Treat it the same way you do foot mange.

NOTE: All species can be attacked by mange, but parakeets are especially susceptible to it.

GOUT

You can readily picture the fat gourmand, his foot reposing on a stool and suffering a thousand martyrdoms, but who refuses to repent for his gluttony.

Well, the frail little bird can also get gout, and for the same reason: he is a little glutton who loves rich food!

You can diagnose this disease very simply: the bird's joints are deformed.

Treat it the way you would any case of gout: by giving the patient less rich food and (if you are "fortunate" enough to have someone in your family who has gout) the same drugs that a human takes but in small doses, of course.

EGG-LAYING TROUBLE

A bird, whether a hen or a canary, lays her eggs betweeen 7 and 8 o'clock in the morning.

If for any reason the female doesn't succeed in expelling the egg, you will find her, when you get up, lying on the floor of the cage exhausted and lacking the strength to even perch. In such an event, grasp her between your fingers as described (see *Handling*, page 233), and squirt several drops of oil into the cloaca; then massage the belly gently.

If this doesn't suffice, this procedure usually induces laying:

(1) While massaging the abdomen gently, coat it with some drops of cooking oil.

(2) Run a thin stream of cold water over the bird's belly for 30 seconds.

(3) Place the bird in a nest containing some cotton that you have previously warmed (77 to 86°F or 25 to 30°C).

(4) To prevent the female from leaving the nest, cover her with some light flannel.

The egg should come out within the next 45 minutes.

Don't forget: When your bird is on the verge of laying, give her some powdered oyster shell or eggshell. In actual fact, without this extra calcium the egg will stay soft and won't be able to come out!

NOTE: Be aware of the fact that any trauma can arrest laying: fright, noise, bright light, etc. Even with your help, an anxious female will not be able to extrude the egg and a vet will have to do . . . a Caesarian!

LIVER DISEASE

The little canary had eaten too many oily seeds (hempseed, rapeseed, etc.). He had a liver attack and it was immediately apparent on him because he was small: he had a dark brown, violaceous spot on his abdomen, about the size of a pea; it was clearly visible if you blew on his feathers.

The same sort of spot is also noticeable on parakeets when they overindulge themselves in egg mash.

It doesn't appear on parrots or other large birds but this doesn't mean that they don't have liver trouble!

Treat the patient in a very simple way:

(1) Alter its diet: cut out the oily seeds or egg mash and replace with canary seed and lettuce seed.

(2) Put Vichy water in its trough and bath.

If after several days of this treatment nothing is improved, obviously it will be necessary to see the vet.

NOTE: Often it's not overeating that is responsible for the liver attack of your little winged friend, but rather . . . yourself!

A "bird in the kitchen" doesn't merely run the risk of getting a head cold: he absorbs the grease of human food through all his pores and usually lacks sufficient oxygen; these factors can suffice to precipitate the crisis. In this event the first thing to do is to put the bird in another room.

THRUSH

This is a fungus that attacks young turtledoves just as it attacks—doubtless you know this—human babies.

You diagnose it because, in birds and babies alike, swallowing is impossible. If you don't take care of your turtledoves right away they won't be able to "break bread" and will starve in the midst of plenty.

So you have to act and act quickly, because thrush spreads rapidly. It is very easy:

(1) Catch the turtledove (see *Handling*, page 233); this is easy because this bird is gentle and semidomesticated.

(2) Open its beak. You will observe that the inside is lined with yellowish, slightly velvety plaques.

(3) Lift off these plaques by means of a pair of tweezers; they come off very easily.

(4) Sprinkle baking soda over the inside of the bird's beak, thus creating an alkaline medium in which the fungus cannot develop. Or, if you don't have baking soda, dab it with iodized glycerine (iodine kills fungi).

(5) Put the bird back in its cage. Normally, it will be cured. Observe it for several days in order to be sure that the fungus doesn't return. If it should return—and that is quite unusual—repeat the same treatment.

(6) Isolate the sick turtledove—which will also allow you to observe it better—and disinfect the aviary: thrush is extremely contagious. Use bicarbonate of soda in a concentration of 2 large tablespoons per pint (about ½ liter) of water.

Don't forget: Thrush is common in turtledoves. If you have one, always keep baking soda or iodized glycerine in your veterinary medicine chest.

MOULTING

All birds moult, and the process almost always causes them suffering.

Moulting is actually a normal biological phenomenon. But beyond this, it bears a close relationship to the animal's sexual life.

Take, for example, those marvelous peacocks that show off by unveiling the splendor of their polychromic tails. Before displaying their royal finery which makes the peahens succumb to their charm, they moult. It is the same for those remarkable egrets, the miniscule and sublime hummingbirds, and, more or less spectacularly, for all other birds.

Now, the avian order—with the exception of nocturnal species—is solar. It is the bright sunlight (more exactly, the lengthening of daylight—*Trans.*) of springtime that stimulates the pituitary gland which, in turn, stimulates the thyroid gland which then stimulates the gonads. An entire chemistry laboratory is thus set in motion, all released by the rays of the sun.

The bird therefore undergoes a veritable and radical physiological crisis, which affects it profoundly and in some cases fatally. That is why you must pay close attention to moulting and treat it as a disease (just as pregnancy is regarded medically as a disease—*Trans.*).

Moulting in canaries

They only moult once, from July to September after reproduction, but the process exhausts them greatly, particularly the females. Anticipate this period of fatigue and take care of your bird if you want it to bear up well. To do so the bird should have:

(1) Very good ventilation.

(2) An enriched diet: add to its food a mixture composed of:

14 ounces (about 400 grams) of oatmeal
7 ounces (about 200 grams) of hempseed
3.5 ounces (about 100 grams) of chicory seeds
3.5 ounces of white lettuce seeds
1.75 ounces (about 50 grams) of Niger seeds
1.75 ounces of poppyseed.

Every other day add to this some chickweed, plantain, grated carrot, apple, and banana.

Lastly, don't forget to give the bird some crushed oyster shell or eggshell, just as at the onset of egg-laying.

(3) Change its water often: a bird needs to drink a lot during moulting. Treatment is the same for all small birds.

Moulting in parakeets

These birds moult two or three times a year, especially if they live in a very warm apartment. Consequently, their moults are more difficult to anticipate than those of a canary. Only by observing them closely can their moults be noticed; but the imperceptibility of their moulting does not make it any less dangerous.

The precautions to take are the same as those for other small birds, except that egg mash should also be added to the food.

Moulting in parrots

An outstanding American ornithologist recommends the following for moulting parrots:

cabbage
wholewheat bread
fresh corn on the cob or, instead, pearl barley
spinach
green onion
pieces of bread soaked in carrot juice, which provides necessary vitamins.

Don't forget to put a piece of sulfur in the bird's drinking water.

Moulting in fledglings

If it is born at the beginning of spring, a bird's first moult takes place at the age of two or three months. However, the bird is actually losing its baby down. True moulting only occurs the following year.

Abnormal moulting

You may have seen those strange canaries or goldfinches whose necks are all covered with feathers that make them look like ridiculous miniature vultures. Well, it's a shortage of sulfur that makes them look so ragged.

The remedy is simple: put a piece of sulfur in the bird's water, and feed it (even a granivore):

(1) Ant eggs (you may have trouble finding an ant hill but they are easy to locate in the country);

(2) Meal worms (get yourself some at a pet shop or at a store where they sell fishing tackle).

French moulting

This is when the bird pulls out its feathers. Classically, this occurs in hybrid degenerates.

It particularly occurs in parrots and parakeets, which plume themselves constantly. It has been known in these birds for a long time. In olden days people were convinced that it stemmed from the fact that the parrot had eaten some meat one day and, trying to recover the taste, pulled out its feathers in order to suck on the ends!

Nothing could be more mistaken.

But the fact is that there are other causes for this renowned condition besides degeneracy. These include an unbalanced diet and sometimes an allergy to the sun and to heat. Often there is a psychosomatic cause: a neglected parrot that doesn't feel like "one of the family" plumes itself as a result of feeling depressed!

Now, contrary to what our grandparents believed, this condition is treated by actually giving the bird some meat! The South African ornithologist Buttner has recommended this meat diet, to which you add some brewer's yeast (a good-sized pinch in the bird's food), some thistle leaves, and some dandelion.

In cases of allergy, keep the bird out of the sun and overheated rooms.

Lastly, speak tenderly to your parrot. Don't forget that he is very sensitive and gets upset if people don't pay attention to him!

Soft moulting

This is a mild but permanent moult. It gives you the impression that the bird's feathery cloak is moth-eaten.

Often, it is a lack of space that is responsible; if so, do provide the bird with a larger cage.

It may also occur because you have forgotten to install a bird-bath; baths are essential for a bird.

But perhaps the bird simply hasn't received enough sunlight.

If none of these factors applies, the condition comes from a dietary insufficiency. If so, put the bird on the normal moulting regimen (see *Abnormal moulting*, page 248) until the moult desists.

Sticky moult

This means that the bird doesn't moult! It's as if its feathers were glued to its body. Also, the moult often begins and then stops short.

Well, this is a psychosomatic disease. Saint Francis of Assisi was right, you see, in thinking of birds as "our little brothers," since, unfortunately for them, they react just as we do!

This abrupt halt takes place either because the little animal is bored or because it is afraid.

This happened to one of my patients, a young canary, who had seen a howling monster suddenly leap in front of its cage: a good, noble hunting dog that certainly didn't mean it any harm— but the bird had never seen one! Out of fright it stopped moulting.

In the case of an arrested moult:

(1) Put the bird in a quiet place and give it as much sunlight as possible.

(2) Give it a rich and varied diet (refer to the appropriate section under *Moulting*).

(3) Make it take . . . Turkish baths! That's right, a steam bath will cure the little bird. For this:

(A) Heat a basin or a large saucepan of water.

(B) Place the cage over it (be careful not to let it fall in, or you will have a boiled bird!).

(C) Cover the cage and the basin in such a way that all the water vapor comes up into the cage.

(D) Use the apparatus for a good 15 minutes.

NOTE: When you remove the cage from the steam bath, be sure not to put it in a cool place; to do so would be to substitute fatal bronchial pneumonia for the sticky moult!

Streaking

This is a false moult; it only attacks fledglings, and for a very simple reason:

You have some little birds several days old and suddenly you notice that their nest is full of down and that they find themselves naked. The first thing that occurs to you is that they have moulted. But it is their parents—brutal birds—who have plumed them. Doubtless they have done so to prepare the nest for the next brood. They remove the mantle of the elder child in order to clothe the baby of the family with it!

This condition can also constitute a perversion of taste. Obviously the fledglings must be separated from their deviant parents and you have to try to raise them yourself. (See *Feeding Fledglings,* page 253.)

NOTE: Before accusing the parents of mistreating their children, check under the fledgling's wings to see if there aren't lice. (See *External Parasites,* page 255.)

MYCOPLASMOSIS

This occurs in bovines—and birds. You can't treat it; only a vet can—and on an emergency basis. I bring it up so that you can recognize it. These are the symptoms:

Wheezing respiration and suffocation.

Actually, just like aspergillosis, at the beginning it resembles pulmonary congestion.

BIRD FALLEN FROM A NEST

The three fledglings started a circus going throughout the house! The three-year-old wolf dog spotted them first. He alerted the family with his yelping and dancing on the lawn. The cat perked up her ears. She leaped through the window and onto a low branch to see—fast. And, being a feline, she crept through the grass.

But the children got there first: three of them, one per fledgling. They returned singing triumphantly, their hands transformed into a nest for each tit. With their new feathers and still-yellow beaks, the little birds were pitiable, trembling after the terrifying adventure that had just befallen them. They opened their beaks as wide as they could in order to cheep and call for help so that Mama Tit would feed them.

The children brought them into the living room and made a nest out of moss in an old pot. But that was all they knew to do. And of course the adults weren't there. So, while two of them kept the cat under observation, who herself was watching the birds with her eyes deceptively half-shut, the most alert child telephoned me to ask my advice.

"Well," I told him, "you and your brothers are going to have something to keep you busy during your vacation! Here is what you are going to do:"

(1) Put the fledglings in a place where it's about 95°F (35°C). As the days go by, gradually decrease the temperature until it gets to 77°F (25°C). (If they have just been born, they are without feathers and are blind; if so, there is no hope of saving them.)

(2) Feed them every 15 minutes, for 6 to 15 days, all day and part of the night (that is, for 18 hours). This is absolutely necessary. To feed them, use an eyedropper, letting the food that they demand fall into their open beaks, drop by drop.

(3) This food consists of a liquid mash that is sold already prepared. You can make it yourself by mixing:

a saltless rusk, ground up into a powder

a thoroughly beaten egg yolk

a pinch of sugar.

Mix the whole thing up with some tepid water (86°F or 30°C) until you get a clear broth.

(4) After 15 days, add some chicory seeds and some dilute milk to the mash. Don't feed them any more frequently than every 30 minutes (still over 18 hours). Keep this up for 7 weeks.

(5) After the seventh week fill the beaks only once an hour.

In the same manner you raise fledglings born in a cage that were orphaned or whose parents abandoned them. This holds for little birds of all species, even insectivores. For the latter, add 2 teaspoons of dried May flies to the mash; and when they are adult, give them meal worms and fresh ant eggs.

Raptorial birds should receive, supplementally, some chopped meat or raw liver, starting from the second week. You also have to get them some rabbit feet and some chicken feathers, chopped up and mixed with sand.

Obviously, the work required to be a bird "nanny" isn't easy. Nevertheless, I have often seen children, aided by their parents, succeed in saving fledglings.

BIRDS IN THE KITCHEN

This isn't meant as instructions on cooking birds but as a warning. People are often inclined to put the bird cage in the kitchen.

This is objectionable for two reasons:

(1) The flavors emanating from a simmering stew aren't at all good for birds; this poisoning can even lead to vision problems and liver damage.

(2) Also harmful are the temperature fluctuations from oven heat. These can range over 27°F (15°C). Furthermore, people then often open the window to air out the kitchen, which results in a cold, pulmonary congestion, etc. for the bird.

FEEDING FLEDGLINGS

Their parents are available, in principle, to feed fledglings. But if the parents happen to die or abandon them (as happens with caged birds), you have to raise the fledglings as if they had fallen from a nest (see *Bird Fallen from a Nest,* page 251).

On the other hand, sometimes you have to improve and enrich the food of the nursing parents. Thus:

Turtledoves and parrots, when they become parents, love to have their ordinary menu supplemented with meal worms and moist bread. This supercharges them and enriches their crop milk, which is a fluid secreted anticipatorily by the crop and which serves to nourish the young.

Be advised that canaries are inconstant parents and are quite prone to abandon their offspring; on the other hand, turtledoves and parrots are very conscientious and never abandon them.

BROKEN LEG

A canary and a Burmese cat of which I have already spoken lived on good terms, the former *in* the cage and the latter *on* the cage, into which the cat tried to stick his paw from time to time. These attempts greatly worried their mistress, who wasn't anxious to see her bird transformed into a succulent meal by and for the Burmese. She was all the more concerned because the happy-go-lucky canary never seemed bothered by that ever-present possibility.

Now, it happened that the bird broke its leg somehow. I was summoned and I made a splint. I recommended that the bird be taken from its cage and placed in a box without crossbars so that the bird wouldn't jump, which would definitely have ruined its leg.

So Mrs. G. put the canary in a cardboard box which she covered with cheesecloth so that the bird wouldn't fly away. Then she placed the box in a room and closed the door carefully so that the cat wouldn't be able to get in.

Several hours passed as she went about her business without being concerned with the matter further. Then she suddenly realized that the Burmese had disappeared. She called to him and then made some noise with his food dish, a sound that he was never able to resist. All was in vain.

"My God," she said with horror, "I shut him up with the bird! Well, no more canary!"

She opened the door. Sure enough, the big cat was purring peacefully, lying up on the table, and against the box—the box where the little bird, relaxed under its friend's watchful eye, was still quite alive.

This happy ending was exceptional, however. If you own a bird and a cat and the former gets sick, I don't advise you to put the cat on duty as a nurse in this manner.

If, however, your canary breaks its leg, here is how to proceed in order to repair it:

(1) If the femur is broken and the fracture isn't open, make a splint with two large matches, making sure that the leg is perfectly straight. Secure the ends of the pieces of wood by winding thread around them, and put the bird in a box so that it can't fly or even walk too much. It takes about 3–5 days for mending to be completed. Then remove the splint and return the bird to its cage.

(2) If it is the tibia that is broken, unfortunately you will have to amputate, for even if you apply a splint very skillfully, the leg will remain askew and will hamper the bird more than if it is an amputee. To do so:

(A) With an assistant, catch and hold the bird.

(B) With a nail clippers, cut the leg at the joint.

(C) Cauterize the wound with a little hydrogen peroxide.

(D) Leave the bird alone in a small cage or box for 48 hours, after which time the amputation should be well healed.

Then return the bird to its cage. You will see that he adjusts very well to his handicap.

EXTERNAL PARASITES

White lice

These infest all birds without exception, from the smallest to the largest, ensconcing themselves in the feathers and living there cosily, finding both food and shelter since they eat the down of the bird. If you blow gently on the bird, you can easily see them: they are big and white. Don't try to de-flea your bird; he's not a cat! Powdered insecticides will rid birds completely of these harmful parasites.

Red lice

Even though they are much smaller than white lice, these have two more legs: eight instead of six. They don't live on the bird but rather approach it at night, taking advantage of its sleep to transform it into a nice steak for lice. Actually, unlike white lice, they suck the bird's blood. During the day they hide in the nest, beneath the roost, or in the corners of the cage.

You have to be careful of them because, in spite of their very small size—⅗ millimeter long—they can cause serious anemia and even death in fledglings.

Since they don't venture out onto the bird during the day, if you examine it then, you won't find them. You can, however, detect their presence because instead of sleeping at night, the canary is restless. In this event, it is best to change its domicile for a day and to wash and disinfect its cage. Use a commercial insecticide that you can buy at a pet store.

NOTE: DDT is dangerous for all animals, feathered as well as furry.

PNEUMONIA

This is the logical sequel of a cold if the latter is not arrested in time. The bird curls up in a ball and breathes with difficulty. It has to be rushed to the vet. If it's a small bird, as I have said, there is no hope, but if it's kind of large (a parrot, for example) it can be given oxygen therapy. This is the only way to save it.

INVERSION OF THE CLOACA

This can take place following two conditions:
(1) Constipation (see *Constipation,* page 240).
(2) The difficulty that a female can have in laying eggs.
The organ called the cloaca is a kind of internal pouch, into which empty the digestive tract, the eggs, and the urinary tract. Under exertion it can turn around and come out. If you will, the bird "has hemorrhoids."

This is easy to detect: it projects under the tail like a big button. But don't be alarmed; you can return it to its normal position very easily. To do so:

(1) Catch and secure the bird (see *Handling,* page 233).
(2) Warm the extruding part with cotton soaked in hot water.

(3) With the aid of a well-oiled *plastic* eyedropper, push the cloaca back into the inside of the bird.

You must then suture the orifice of the cloaca with stitches referred to as the Valsalva purse. A woman will know how to do this very well: you make several stitches around the opening and draw them loosely because they have to be gathered.

Remove the thread after 48 hours.

REPRODUCTION

NOTE: The reproductive instinct can be abolished in the bird if its environment does not correspond to that which it would have in nature.

So as soon as it reaches courting age, think about offering it a nest, along with some little scraps of wool so that it can fix up and personalize your prefab nest.

Lighting is also very important. Thus birds that are condemned to live in artificial light never reproduce.

If you want to have fledglings, the future parents must have sunlight. The sun's bright, warm rays arouse their desire to reproduce.

In addition, the temperature of the cage should never drop below 59°F (15°C).

CUTTING THE NAILS

Particularly in the canary, the nail grows out and curves back on itself, preventing the bird from perching since it can no longer grasp the bars. You can diagnose this very easily: the bird remains on the floor of its cage. In such a case:

(1) Get someone to help you and then catch the bird (see *Handling,* page 233).

(2) Hold the foot in your left hand and examine it. You can easily see the rosy digit in its horny sheath.

(3) With a nail clippers cut the claw about $\frac{1}{12}$ inch (2 millimeters) down.

(4) If by accident you cut too high and the toe bleeds, stop the bleeding immediately with a little hydrogen peroxide.

SWEATING

One day I was called by a client who said to me:

"My canary is perspiring so, that its wings look as if they were smeared with birdlime."

"Might your canary be a female and might she not have fledglings?"

She was astonished. "How did you know that?"

I was no sorcerer; what is described as "sweating" in a bird is due to the fact that its young have diarrhea so liquid that the bird patrols everywhere but never succeeds in disposing of it all. (For the first seven days of their life, their mother consumes their droppings.) And when she tries to dry off her beak on her feathers, she has to start all over again—which gives the impression that she is "sweating."

Fledglings that contract this enteritis generally die from it very rapidly. You can take them to the vet and have him try antibiotics. As for the mother, you have to catch her (see *Handling*, page 233) and wash her with a wad of cotton moistened with warm water.

GAPEWORM INFECTION

This is referred to in books on falconry as threadworm, but the man in the street knows it by the descriptive term "bucket beak," which expresses well what it means. The bird that contracts it actually yawns constantly.

This strange disease is due to an unusual worm that is shaped like a Y, and for a very unseemly reason: it actually consists of two worms, a male and a female, which love unites for the duration of their lives!

The earthworm is the host of this erotic "Y," or, more accurately, of its eggs. So when a bird eats earthworms, it can develop gapeworm infection.

Moral: if you have some insectivorous birds (magpies, crows, raptorial species, pheasants, etc.) in an aviary, avoid giving them earthworms.

VOMITING

Don't confuse this with the normal regurgitation of food for their fledglings, which occurs in numerous species of birds from the eagle to the pigeon.

I have personally never seen a bird vomit, but several breeders have assured me that this sometimes happens to overfed parrots.

In such an event, dissolve 3 or 4 granules of soda citrate in the bird's drinking water and put it on half rations for one or two days.

NOTE: I *mean* half rations. On a full diet, he will die from thi⁓

► WILD BIRDS

One more often has small birds than large ones in a cage or aviary. However, you may have to take care of a big bird. You may own one, or you may have found one out in the country, fallen from its nest and injured, or abandoned (which happens, for example, on migratory flights: the birds of the last brood, being too young, cannot follow along). So you should know how to administer first aid in such a situation.

I have already instructed you, under *Handling* (see page 233), how to hold them in order to minister to them. I emphasize that, if you have to deal with raptorial birds, you can never be too careful of their claws, which are even more dangerous than their beaks.

Here, then, are the main types of emergency.

BROKEN WING (OR LEG)

A wine grower of Ribeauvillé in Alsace told me this remarkable story.

"This was when there were still storks in Alsace, about 20 years ago. I was walking in the woods with my wife when, in a clearing, an astonishing spectacle petrified us. In this rather spacious area, which looked like a city square in the middle of the trees, several hundred storks were assembled. Apparently they hadn't seen us and, hiding behind some bushes, we were able to observe them at play.

"At first, we couldn't figure anything out. They squawked, cheeped, and seemed very busy. From time to time one of them would fly up in the air while all the others watched; and then, sooner or later, it would come to rest again among the others.

"Finally we grasped the meaning of this assembly: the storks were going to migrate and before the great departure, they were making the year-old fledglings take test flights in order to see which of them were capable of leaving along with the others.

"Each young stork circled overhead several times and then returned. The older birds would peck at it with their beaks in order to force it to keep flying, since they had to be sure that it would be able to cover the hundreds, indeed thousands of miles which separated the birds from the location where they were going to spend the winter. After four or five laps, some of the fledglings were exhausted and weren't able to take off again.

"So my wife and I witnessed a horrible scene—or at least one that appeared so to our human sensibilities. But doubtless the storks were right in what they were doing. With beak blows directed at its head, they killed each fledgling that couldn't stay airborne long enough. But the bird would have died of exhaustion along the route anyway; they were thus saving it from prolonged suffering."

I myself was familiar with these southward migratory flights by storks, when I was in Morocco. Returning home one evening, I found a young stork caught in the telegraph wires. It had broken a leg and lay motionless on the ground. It gazed toward the sky as if it could still make out its flock, the members of which had ignored its fall and had continued their flight inexorably toward their destination in Chad.

I picked up the bird and performed an osteosynthesis, just like for a human (see page 266). This, I hasten to add, is a matter solely for the vet.

So if you ever come across a stork, a flamingo, an eaglet, or an owl with a broken leg or wing, you can only do two things for it:

(1) Disinfect the wound with hydrogen peroxide.
(2) Prevent it from flying (see *Handling*, page 233).

Next, and as quickly as possible, carry it to the vet.
After the operation, my young stork recovered very well. While

waiting for it to be able to resume its flight, I had installed it in a large cage. Everything seemed to be going for the better when, about a month after its accident, I found it dead one morning.

Why? There was no apparent medical reason.

By and by, at each bird migration, the same thing happened. I found an injured bird, cared for it, cured it—and it died! Was it from sadness at being isolated from its flock? From boredom? Loneliness? I don't know.

If the same problem presents itself to you, maybe you will have better luck than I . . . but don't count on it.

On the other hand, the crow and the magpie adjust very well to being separated from their fellows. Lacking a gregarious instinct, they are easily tamed (especially the crow) and get along amicably with man. If they have a broken wing or leg, treat it as instructed (see *Broken Wing*, page 236; and *Broken Leg*, page 254). If they have fallen from their nest, begin by feeding them like any other bird with artificial crop milk (see *Bird Fallen from a Nest*, page 251). Soon after, add chopped meat to that. From the second week onwards give them the following mash:

2 teaspoons of paste for insectivores (sold already prepared at pet shops)
2 pinches of chopped raw meat
1 chopped hard-boiled egg yolk
1 pinch of chopped carrot.

Some advice: if you have cats, regardless of their apparent behavior, be wary of their reaction. They aren't all little saints; the Burmese whose story I recounted to you was an exception.

I had a client who owned about twenty cats and a dog . . . and a crow. They all lived in the same room and, to all appearances, on good terms, the cats on the floor and the bird perched near the ceiling. Doubtless my client believed that she had raised Noah's ark, and in fact the cats never made a move to pounce on the crow; they seemed to ignore it totally.

They lived together for several years like that, when one day their mistress returned home carrying a bag containing the crow's food. Unfortunately the bag broke open and the food fell on the floor. Mr. Crow, tantalized by the smell, had the bad luck to descend from his perch. No sooner had he reached the floor than the twenty cats swooped down on him. After a few seconds, nothing more than a feather remained of him.

COMMON COLD

See *Common Cold* under Parrots, page 266.

DIGESTIVE TROUBLES

See *Intestinal Troubles* under Parrots, page 268.

INTESTINAL TROUBLES

See *Intestinal Troubles* under Parrots, page 268.

⌐ PARROTS

These beautiful birds, excellent talkers, occupy a place apart because they can talk, of course, which is always astonishing, but also because, unlike most birds, they can be tamed admirably.

Parakeets, macaws, and cockatoos are cared for in the same manner as parrots.

SHARPENING THE BEAK

Although a cuttlefish bone suffices for sharpening a canary's beak, it is not adequate for a parakeet (which, moreover, often refuses to use it) and still less for a parrot.

If it doesn't get sharpened naturally, the horny upper part of the beak grows outward and eventually becomes so prominent that it interferes with the bird's eating. Therefore it is up to you to sharpen it. To do so:

(1) If it's a small bird (a parakeet), put it in a cardboard tube for the operation (see *Handling*, page 233). If it's a large bird (parrot or macaw), you'll need someone to help you. Wearing gloves, your assistant grasps the bird as I have described (see *Handling*), and also holds the beak so as not to be bitten. NOTE: The bird is in a very bad mood and is disposed to vent its anger on the first finger that it can get hold of.

(2) Take a razor blade or lancet and chip away a little of the thin, horny layers until the beak is sufficiently sharpened.

FEEDING OF THE YOUNG BIRDS

(See also *Reproduction,* page 257.)

Sometimes a parrot is born in a cage. (In parakeets this is the usual case, but they are excellent parents and there is almost never any problem. See *Streaking,* page 251.)

Now, if the mother refuses to feed the fledgling or if she dies, it is up to you to raise the orphaned or abandoned parrot.

In such a situation this is what an American ornithologist recommends for the first ten days. Mix:

6 teaspoons of wheat germ
2 fresh egg yolks
½ teaspoon table salt
½ teaspoon ground cuttlefish bone
vitamins: the dose for a nurseling.

Make a broth out of this mixture, mix in some milk, and give it to the little parakeet, divided over four meals per day.

The "nurseling" must remain in the nest for two or three months, so continue to feed it, gradually adding some sunflower seeds, peanuts, walnuts, and crushed hazelnuts to the preceding mash.

BROKEN WING

One day, the macaw belonging to some of my friends had . . . an auto accident!

Its owner, a bird dealer, has a shop not far from my office. The macaw is deep blue, truly one of the most beautiful birds that I have seen, and at the same time very gentle (unlike the "soldier" kind, which are mean). It is so tame that it is allowed to go free in the shop.

Some time ago, the macaw found the door open and decided to go outside for some air. It fluttered out into the middle of the street amidst the traffic and a car struck it, breaking its wing.

Several minutes later the macaw and its owner, both quite upset, entered my office.

I performed an osteosynthesis which succeeded very well (osteosynthesis is an operation which consists of reinforcing the broken bone with an electrically neutral steel pin).

The macaw has resumed its place in the shop. It no longer ventures out into the street.

Quite frequently a parrot, a cockatoo, or a macaw breaks a wing, especially if it flies around freely. The reason is very simple: the feathers on one side of the bird have been deliberately clipped in order to unbalance it and prevent it from flying away. Fluttering about clumsily, it runs into something or else takes a bad fall.

Above all, don't decide to treat this kind of fracture yourself: a parrot is not a canary. An osteosynthesis must be performed and the bird will usually respond quite well, but only a vet is capable of this operation. Confine yourself to giving the bird first aid (see *Broken Wing* (*or Leg*) under Wild Birds, page 260) and carry it to its doctor as fast as possible.

COMMON COLD

My feathered friend Jacotte is from Gabon. She is talkative but a little shy, and a tease. Her master is an important governmental representative and is thin, engaging, and a little nuts. They have the same mischievous eyes and understand each other wonderfully well.

One autumn he, his wife, children, and parrot were out in the country when Jacotte, until then peacefully perched on her master's finger, felt the urge to fly up on the lowest branch of a tree. She selected the biggest tree around for this mission.

When she had reached it, she called "good-bye" mockingly to her family and began to climb farther up the trunk.

No one was very concerned since the family was used to her fantasies—that is, until she was called but flatly refused to come down.

Night came and the children were worried. The government official set the highest ladder available against the tree and valiantly went in pursuit of the bird. Jacotte found this very entertaining, for as her master climbed up each succeeding step, she climbed from branch to branch ahead of him. The ladder only extended one-third of the way up the tree, so he had to give up hope of overtaking her.

"Bah!" he snorted. "She'll come down tomorrow morning when she gets hungry."

But Jacotte did not come down. The first few days she remained in the garden, refusing to return but chatting casually with the family. Then one morning no one heard her any more.

Each of them imagined, without saying so out loud, that a cat or else hunger had finally decided her fate. All eyes were red from crying.

Nevertheless, she was spoken about once more one evening. The official, who is also the mayor of his village, saw a farmer approach. The man, who was frightened blurted out unceremoniously:

"There is a ghost in the yew tree at the cemetery—the tree has started talking!"

No doubt Jacotte was playing the part of the ghost. The official reassured the villager and set out, with him, to try to capture her. But she had already taken off.

Dreary days passed and it became necessary to admit that the parrot had definitely disappeared.

One evening a storm broke, violently announcing the end of the summer. The official and his children, their noses pressed against the windows, pretended to watch the branches bending before the assault of the wind and rain. In fact they were thinking of Jacotte.

Then suddenly, between two thunder claps, a desperate voice was heard crying:

"Papa, I'm cold! Mama, I'm hungry, I'm hungry!"

And a ragged ball, its feathers plastered down, threw itself down before the door, whining in a high, piercing voice.

You can imagine how quickly the door was opened. Jacotte entered the house, glared angrily at everyone whom she deemed responsible for her state, and with a final "Mama, I'm hungry," hurried over to her feeder.

Don't think that I am making this up or exaggerating; the story is authentic to the least detail.

As there is a God, Jacotte was punished for her escapade. The next morning she began to scratch her ears and then to sneeze. She had caught a cold.

Her master went to the medicine cabinet for the bottle of vaseline oil that had recently been used on the youngest child. He put a drop in each of Jacotte's nostrils while she choked with anger. A fine way to treat a Prodigal Son! With several heartfelt oaths, she declared with a nasal voice that she would remember this!

But that didn't stop her master from continuing the treatment, twice a day, until she was cured.

And that is what I advise you to do if your parrot catches cold.

You can also care for it by giving it a Turkish bath (see *Sticky moult*, page 250) in which are placed several eucalyptus leaves.

LARYNGO-TRACHEITIS

One day Jacotte tried hard to say "Good morning," but her voice was so hoarse that she could only emit some rattling noises, much to her consternation. On top of that, she began to yawn to such an extent that her human family noticed.

In a bad mood, she puffed up her feathers and closed her eyes. There was no mistaking it: following the cold she had had the week before, she had developed laryngo-tracheitis. Her human "father" went to get the whiskey bottle.

Fifteen drops in a tablespoon of water gave Jacotte the greatest feeling—she was unsteady but sprightly on her feet— and did her a great deal of good. A little honey in her drinking water finished the job of fixing her up.

There is no better medication against laryngo-tracheitis in a parrot.

INTESTINAL TROUBLES

Give the patient 5 or 6 drops of paregoric elixer, directly into the beak, and sprinkle its food with bismuth subnitrate (see *Constipation*, page 240; and *Diarrhea*, page 242).

► FISH

It mustn't be forgotten that fish disease isn't individual but collective. When a fish gets sick, usually it is the ambient milieu that must be treated, much more than the individual.

The first thing to know is that when you buy a new fish, you have to quarantine it for 10 to 15 days; thus if it carries germs, it won't contaminate the whole aquarium. You must do the same thing—and immediately—when you notice that a fish is diseased.

So if you have a large aquarium, keep a smaller one at its side for newcomers and sick fish. It will also be useful for reproduction, since the majority of fish readily devour their offspring.

The aquarium is a self-enclosed world which can be sufficient unto itself—as long as everything works perfectly. Sometimes, however, this smooth functioning is interrupted by a technical problem.

Thus it was that one of my clients telephoned me one day:

"Doctor, there is a power shortage. I just phoned the electric company and they cannot tell me when the electricity will be restored, but it will take at least several hours. By then, my fish will be dead—you know that I have some very delicate species. What should I do?"

His problem was more a matter for an electrician than for me. But sometimes a little common sense is enough to mitigate a catastrophe.

"Take the battery out of your car. . . ."

He hesitated a second and then understood:

"That's the solution! I connect it up. . . ."

269

That's right, most aquaria run on 6 volts (which is why they are equipped with a transformer). Therefore, a car battery can keep them going in the event of a power breakdown.

Don't forget this may save the lives of your fish!

HOW TO CARE FOR A FISH

If a fish is sick, you have to catch it, either with your hand or with the aid of a little scoop, and isolate it in an aquarium hospital where you will treat it. This treatment generally (except where an injury is concerned) consists of baths:

Occupying first place among the fish's friends is coarse, grey sea salt (see *Medicine Chest for Fish*, page 281). Right behind this comes methylene blue (again see *Medicine Chest*), which has only one drawback: it colors the aquarium sand grey.

When there is a wound or ulcer, remove the fish from the aquarium and, holding it in one hand, paint the affected area with mercurochrome using the other hand. Obviously you have to work fast: the patient doesn't appreciate the terrestrial atmosphere.

Potassium permanganate is also an excellent remedy (see *Medicine Chest*).

Finally, if you have to disinfect the aquarium, first lift the fish out and then clean its habitat with a copper sulfate solution (see *Copper sulfate*, page 282).

BACTERIA

These attack cyprinoids in particular (including goldfish) but are only found in water polluted by organic material. The precautions to take and the treatment to give are the same: see to it that the aquarium is clean.

PARASITIC FUNGI

These infest wounds which are either of parasitic origin or caused by fights or injuries. The skin, gills, and fins appear to be covered with soap lather.

You have a choice of three medications:

(1) Salt bath: ¼ ounce (7 grams) per quart (liter) of water, for 30 minutes.

(2) Potassium permanganate bath: 100 cubic centimeters of a 1% solution per liter of water, for 30 minutes.

(3) Collargol bath: .000001 per liter of water for 20 minutes.

NOTE: Do not exceed the doses or times indicated.

Then isolate the patient for a week, placing it in very pure and aerated water at a temperature about 3½°F (2°C) above its accustomed milieu.

CONSTIPATION

Except for goldfish, which are very prone to this, fish only get constipated because they are too well fed.

This condition is readily apparent: the excrement is hard, calcareous, and sparse.

The remedy is that used for man: castor oil.

If the fish is rather large, administer 2 drops directly with an eye-dropper, taking advantage of a moment when it opens its mouth to breathe.

If the fish is too small for this, dunk a worm in the oil and offer it to the patient by means of a pair of tweezers.

Next step: a balanced diet.

HEATSTROKE

This can occur naturally in very warm climates or may be due to a mechanical accident. It causes asphyxia in the fish because the dissolved oxygen that fish breathe is dissipated. The water must be cooled as rapidly as possible and yet gradually, or else there is a risk of hemolysis (see *Hemolysis,* page 276).

CHILLING

If the aquarium water is too cold, the fish grows pale, its fins get plastered against its body, and it becomes vulnerable to parasites and fungi.

Warm the water gradually and then maintain it at 2 or 3°F (1 or 2°C) above the normal temperature for a week. In addition, make the water slightly salty (⅓ ounce, or 10 grams, per quart of water).

FATTY DEGENERATION

If too well fed, the little red fish becomes fat, lazy, slow, and soft. It should be treated as though it had enteritis (see *Enteritis*, page 275) and then given a balanced diet. Ask your pet store owner to recommend one.

WATER

As I have said, it is more important to take care of its water than the fish itself. Now, the first indication of an imbalance in this biological equilibrium is a change, to some extent in the color of the water, which is normally always very clear.

In the water live not only the fish but also plants which are indispensable to them, constituting part of their food (especially the algae) but above all furnishing the oxygen which the fish need.

You can tell that the water is healthy from the fact that:

(1) It is clear.
(2) The rocks at the bottom of the aquarium are partly covered with green algae, forming a kind of gelatinous moss.

If the algae become yellow or brown, this is an indication of a lack of light. If they become pale sea-green, this means that there is too much light. (You know, of course, that an aquarium should receive seven hours of light per day.)

Green water

One of my colleagues, who has an aquarium, left for a vacation. So that his fish would have enough but not too much light, he put them in front of the window, relying on the diurnal rhythm of sunlight to maintain a normal environment.

When he returned home, green algae had invaded the entire bottom of the aquarium, to the point where the water had become green from them: they had received too much light. The green water isn't actually unhealthy in itself, but it makes the algae vulnerable to the slightest change in the weather. If there is a storm or merely a hot day, the algae die and the water then becomes a culture medium for bacteria.

Therefore, it is essential to prevent the algae from invading the whole aquarium. To do so:

(1) First of all, there is preventive treatment: limiting the lighting—which isn't always easy when you're not there! So if you go away, give your keys to someone who will be able to adjust the light.

(2) If despite these precautions the water turns green, put blue paint on the side of the aquarium facing the light.

(3) If the algae have become way too abundant, set the aquarium in total darkness for 48 hours. The algae will disappear.

(4) If this still doesn't do the job, buy some colonies of live Daphnia and put them in the aquarium. They will be delighted with the green aquatic pastures at their disposal.

(5) A last solution: acidify the water by adding several drops of acidic sodium phosphate (ready-made solutions of this are at pet stores).

Brown water

This is much more dangerous than green water, of which it is the converse: its color is due to the proliferation of yellow and brown algae, which only develop in shade and which are poisonous to certain fish.

To combat it:

(1) Preventive treatment: light! This brown water is only encountered in dark rooms where the aquarium is poorly illuminated.

(2) If the algae aren't abundant, they can be removed with a scraper and a siphon.

(3) If the algae are copious, eliminate them by washing the aquarium with a solution of potassium permanganate or of copper sulfate (if you use the latter, it obviously is necessary to first remove the fish). (See *Medicine Chest for Fish,* page 281.) Then disseminate some more green algae.

(4) Lastly, see to it that somehow the aquarium has sufficient light (I reiterate: seven hours per day) so that the problem does not recur.

Milky water

The water first becomes greyish and then milky. The fault lies completely with owners of aquaria who, like dog or bird owners, give their pets too much to eat.

The overabundant food breaks up in the water. This is very serious because the water can and does become filled with bacteria and other micro-organisms that will flourish there.

In such an event:

(1) Don't give the fish anything to eat for 48 hours; they will then be forced to clean the water in order to eat!

(2) Change half of the water, then add to the aquarium a solution of potassium permanganate (see *Potassium permanganate,* page 282).

(3) If this isn't sufficient, remove the fish and wash the bottom of the aquarium with a copper sulfate solution (see *Copper sulfate,* page 282).

Flaky water

A kind of deposit collects on the bottom of the aquarium, taking the form of flakes. No one knows its cause but it often establishes itself in aquaria where there live fish that are big eaters and big consumers of oxygen.

In this case you treat only the water . . . with water! Replace about 20% of it with fresh water and repeat several days later. Keep this up until the flakes have all disappeared.

Cloudy water

This is due to a problem with the filter.

Lastly, I caution you that if the plants in the water become sickly, this indicates that your aquarium is sick. It is up to you, or the vet, to determine its illness.

Don't forget: Just as fish don't all like the same things to eat, the temperature and acidity of the water vary according to the species. So only put fish together that have the same tastes.

GAS BUBBLES

This condition is caused by excessive oxygenation of the water. In most cases, the plants are too abundant and the light is too bright.

As soon as you notice this, place the fish in neutral water that is normally oxygenated.

ENTERITIS

The excrement is yellow and mucoid, the pigmentation of the body darkens. . . .

This is the disease of the overly well-nourished fish. Treat it as you would for an obese human: put the fish on a diet—and for a long time, from 5 to 15 days.

In addition, avoid giving it breadcrumbs or spoiled meat; these can precipitate enteritis.

PARASITIC FLAGELLATES

These .01-millimeter organisms attack fish that are already weakened.

The fish moves ahead jerkily, its fins are plastered against its body, and its skin takes on a bluish-white cast.

Every other day, bathe the fish in a solution of 1 ounce (about 30 grams) of table salt per quart (liter) of water, for 15 minutes.

Disinfect the aquarium, of course.

HEMOLYSIS

This is the destruction of red blood cells. It results from an abrupt change of temperature in the ambient water. Whole aquaria have died from this, following a prolonged power failure. There is nothing that can be done to save the residents.

HYDRAS

One of my clients who lived out in the country phoned me one day, perplexed:

"I happen to have some young fish and they have all disappeared. What disease attacked them?"

"None, to be sure. Are you certain that neither their father nor their mother has eaten them?"

"Positive! They are very timid cichlids—*Apistogramma*—and, as you know, they never eat their young."

"In that case, you have hydras!"

"Yes I do, in fact."

"Don't look any further: it is they that are responsible. In order to get rid of them, empty your aquarium and clean it with a solution of copper sulfate." (See *Copper sulfate*, page 282.)

The hydra is a gentle little aquatic polyp of about ½ inch (1 centimeter) in length whose shape vaguely resembles that of the mythological Hydra, hence its name.

It fastens itself against the side of the aquarium or under a rock, and it waits there patiently to see what happens along that it can snap up. Its favorite tidbit is young fish.

These hydras are only found in stocked aquaria, not in city water. But they are also found in well water and reservoir water, which is where my client's aquarium got them, evidently.

NOTE: If you have hydras in your aquarium, don't slice them in half when you remove them. If you do, you'll have as many hydras as pieces!

PARASITIC CILIATES

Imagine a frightening world, somewhere in an unknown galaxy, where each being lives for no more than 50 hours but gives rise to a thousand offspring—isn't that scary?

Such a world actually exists among the infinitely tiny organisms: it is that of the infusorians. And their thousands of young attack fish in order to live. Their presence is easily detected: numerous white points appear on the skin and the fins.

The affected fish should immediately be put in a quinine bath (1 gram of quinine sulfate per quart of water) and left there until the white spots disappear, which sometimes takes 20 days.

Take advantage of the occasion to wash the aquarium and to disinfect it with methylene blue (several drops per quart of water). Change the water once a day for a week.

LINGERING ILLNESS

Alone all day without any friends, the little fish was bored. In the evening when Man came home from work, he found the fish pressed against the side of its aquarium, frisking about with joy at his return. But the fish was so gloomy during the day that it forgot to eat. It was as though its loneliness was so oppressive that it preferred to die—which sometimes does happen!

So Man gave the fish some friends. It was so happy that its neurosis disappeared.

Don't forget: Just like a bird, a fish that is left alone in a room where it cannot see anyone gets upset and may die.

PARASITIC DISEASES

Fish louse

If you see a little fish rubbing against the rocks in its aquarium, it is scratching itself. And it is scratching itself because it has just been bitten—just as you get bitten by a mosquito—by a crustacean 4 millimeters long: the fish louse. This is a fish "vampire" which bites fish in order to feed on their blood.

They are easily seen with a magnifying glass. You have to:

Remove the fish from the water and pull off the parasite. Then submerge the patient for 15 seconds in a bath of 2% lysol.

NOTE: Once you detect the presence of this organism, you must empty the whole aquarium and wash it meticulously.

Ergasilus

These tiny, 1.5-millimeter crustaceans consist almost entirely of a pair of pincers, by means of which they hang onto the fish's gills. They tear into the tissue, thus causing a respiratory disease which almost always kills the fish.

Try to save the patient by plunging it into a bath of salt water (1 ounce or 30 grams of salt per quart) and forcing it to swim around in it.

Lemacocera

The red fish had something like a long white thread coming out of its gill. This meant that the female of a parasite, *Lemacocera*, had attached itself to the fish in order to lay its eggs there.

This is serious because once the eggs are laid, the *Lemacocera* dies and falls off, leaving the fish with a little wound through which fungi or bacteria can enter.

In such a case:

(1) Isolate the fish.

(2) As soon as the parasite comes off, dip the patient in a bath made up of ¼ ounce (7 grams) of table salt per quart (liter) of water.

(3) Every 12 hours add 2 grams of salt to this. The bath must be continued for 36 hours in all.

(4) Next place the fish under observation for 4 or 5 days, in water containing 5 grams of salt per liter of water.

(5) If all goes well, put the fish back in the aquarium.

LACK OF AERATION

You've seen the fishbowl with red fish—you know, these round fishbowls, usually set on top of something and in which a red fish swims around untiringly.

I even disliked them when I was a child. An old friend of my mother had one in which, like clockwork, a red fish would die and would be replaced immediately by another one, while the old woman complained that "These store owners are dishonest; they sell me sick fish. This latest one is already dead."

In order to keep me out of mischief, she would set me in front of the cyprinoid and tell me: "Watch the little fish."

I was hypnotized by that prisoner and I would have given anything to set it free. Thus it was that I made an accidental movement and broke its glass prison. I am convinced that, without wanting to do so consciously, I somehow did it intentionally.

The atrocious "fishbowl with red fish" also represents a monstrous mistake, for the fish lacks air in there and may die. Contrary to what is often believed, a fish does not transform water into oxygen and hydrogen. In order to breathe, it must have oxygen dissolved in its water. (This, of course, explains the importance of plants in an aquarium.)

For a cyprinoid to be able to survive in a fishbowl, the latter must only be ⅔ filled with water. This leaves a cushion of air sufficient to allow the little fish to breathe. The well-meaning woman of my childhood filled the fishbowl to the brim, convinced that this would please her little captive. But the result was death—by asphyxia.

LACK OF OXYGEN

This is due to poor aeration or to an overpopulated aquarium.

The fish remain on the surface, opening and closing their mouths nervously.

Give them oxygen at once, if you don't want them to die.

PLANARIANS

These are flatworms, about ¾ inch (20 millimeters) long, which have exactly the same bad habits as hydras (see *Hydras*, page 276). You will have a great deal of trouble getting rid of them because they are resistant to all disinfectants.

The best remedy—not to say the only one—is to put a fish called *Trichogaster tricopterus*, or the blue gourami, in the aquarium. It loves planarians—in the most voracious manner!

PRECAUTIONS TO TAKE

Even more important than treating fish attacked by parasites is preventing the latter from taking up residence in an aquarium. To do so:

(1) As soon as you have detected a case of disease, isolate the sick fish and meticulously disinfect the aquarium.

(2) Only use riverbed sand in an aquarium after letting it dry out for several months (if it is you who have collected it).

(3) Keep the aquarium water clean at all times.

(4) Disinfect whatever wounds the fish may sustain.

(5) Never introduce any fish with damaged fins into an aquarium.

(6) Last and most important, learn to know your fish. If one of them gets sick you should be able to notice this immediately.

RICKETS

This stems from artificial food that is low in vitamins. The appearance of the skin changes, and the fins begin to fall apart. A fish in this condition should be given live prey, or else little pieces of very fresh chopped meat.

WORMS

There are many kinds of these worms, but only some of them are dangerous, let alone frequently fatal. Principal among these are:

Gyrodactyls, which especially attack sailfish. You detect this condition by the fact that the fish "scratches itself" against every object that it comes across, and the gills remain open. When you remove the fish from the water, you notice that its body is covered with mucus.

You should quickly isolate the fish and give it an ammonia bath (10% per quart of water) for 15 minutes, repeating this once daily for four days.

Thoroughly disinfect the aquarium.

MEDICINE CHEST FOR FISH

Coarse sea salt

This is a panacea for fish diseases. It contains sodium chloride, obviously, but it also contains all the nutrients that they need.

NOTE: I mean coarse grey salt, not refined salt.

The classical concentration is 5 grams per liter of water plus 1 supplementary gram every 6 hours, up to 10 grams per liter. But you can exceed this guideline in certain cases.

Methylene blue

This is an extraordinary disinfectant. It is applied in 5% aqueous solution, in a concentration of 2 drops of this solution per liter of water. This stuff is a big inconvenience, however, since the aquarium becomes dull: the sand and rocks turn greyish.

Mercurochrome

This is used especially for wounds and ulcers. It is applied in 10% aqueous solution, at a concentration of one drop per liter of water. When it is used preventively for a disinfectant bath, the concentration is 3 drops per 10 liters of water.

Bear in mind that plants are easily harmed by coarse salt and by methylene blue, but they are not very sensitive to mercurochrome.

Potassium permanganate

This is an antiseptic beloved by aquarium lovers. It acts principally through its remarkable oxydizing properties. It is employed in the following manner:

(1) Prepare a solution of 4 grams of permanganate dissolved in a liter of water.

(2) Prepare a medicinal bath in a small aquarium hospital by putting 4 dessert spoons (40 milliliters) of the above solution into 10 liters of water.

(3) Immerse the sick fish in this bath for 30 minutes (except for Japanese ricefish, which can only stand 15 minutes).

This treatment should be repeated every other day until healing is complete.

The concentrated solution is used only to treat wounds by direct application.

Potassium permanganate is also employed as a disinfectant for contaminated objects. The dose for this purpose is 1 gram per 100 liters of water.

Copper sulfate

Blue vitriol, "the friend of the horse's foot," is also used on fish, but *note* that it is extremely toxic. You must therefore observe the patient's reactions closely because they may very well be adverse.

Two techniques are of value:

(1) Baths of from 10 to 15 minutes—no longer—at a dose of 1 gram per 10 liters of water.

(2) Putting 4 teaspoons (20 milliliters) of a 1:1000 solution of

copper sulfate in 10 liters of water. You can then leave patients in this bath for about 12 days, since it is much less dangerous than the preceding one.

Lastly, a tried-and-true technique consists of decorating the bottom of the aquarium with a piece of red copper (a couple of inches of electrical cord from which the insulation has been scraped and which is scrunched up into a ball works just as well). In order to convert the copper into a soluble, active salt, all you have to do next is to add either some 1:100 sea water or else a pinch of sea salt per liter of water to the aquarium.

▸REPTILES AND AMPHIBIANS

I used to know Cleopatra—but I don't mean that I was Marc Antony in a former life. Cleopatra was a charming—oh, how charming—snake who adored her young mistress and showed her affection by twisting around her neck or arm. Thus, the girl could take her to high school hidden under a collar or sleeve.

All sorts of activities whirled around Cleo: she was "borrowed" for use in solving a geometry problem, or for representing the map of France. But if her mistress displeased her, the snake would slip to the floor. One day, for example, Cleo slithered across the feet of the Latin teacher—which brought the lesson to an abrupt end!

I once knew the prominent director of an important professional society who liked animals so much that he had a couple of young crocodiles in his bathtub. He also had a boa constrictor that died and received this funeral oration: "Boas certainly aren't very hardy. Next time I'm going to buy a python." And he did!

Regarding unusual pets, I once knew of a tortoise that weighed over 30 pounds. It loved to tease people—it wedged itself behind the door to its owners' apartment like a big rock, thus preventing them from getting back in.

I made the tortoise's acquaintance at the veterinary school of Toulouse where, following the completion of my studies, I was a professor's assistant. A young student brought the tortoise to me and, pointing out a swelling on the animal's leg, gave me his diagnosis:

"It's a tumor!"

I examined and palpated the lesion.

"I would say it's an abscess."

"Oh, no, sir," he said respectfully. "Abscesses are warm."

He had forgotten that the tortoise is a cold-blooded animal. It was, in fact, a cold abscess into which I made my incision.

On the other hand, tortoises generally take pretty good care of themselves. Another one that I had for a customer had her shell broken by a dog. But the dog had an excuse: he was under the impression that the tortoise was a big rock. That this rock should suddenly start walking drove him crazy. A rock that thinks it can walk? I'll show it!

I bandaged Madame Tortoise's wounds, glued her shell back together, and returned her to the garden, where the dog no longer dared touch her once he understood that this rock was alive.

I am telling you all this in order to emphasize that the most unusual animals, even snakes—which strike fear into most people—can become household pets. If they get sick, see a vet rather than try to treat them yourself. I shall give you some advice: choose a zoo veterinarian, who will be qualified to take care of the kind of animal that you possess. City and country vets aren't trained to be familiar with iguanas or rattlesnakes.

Furthermore, it is rare for a snake to be sick—except for indigestion. The same is true of lizards and chameleons. Tortoises, on the other hand, are accident-prone but can be treated quite successfully, as I have just illustrated.

Whatever animal you have adopted, from the ordinary cat or dog to the strange mongoose, the dangerous panther, or the scary snake, don't forget that the first thing to do to maintain its health is to keep it happy. If it behaves as though you will want to throw it out after several days like a broken toy, don't take it. Even if well nourished and cared for, it will fall ill and may even let itself die of boredom or depression—and all the more readily, the closer it is to the wild state.

► THE BEHAVIOR OF DOMESTIC ANIMALS

A domestic animal is one that has been bred by man; that is, man has exerted sufficient control over its evolution to render the animal significantly different from its wild ancestor. This difference between domestic and wild animals, then, is genetic. A dog, for example, represents a distinct species from its ancestor, the wolf (even though the two animals can interbreed). The reason for these genetic differences is, of course, that the two animals have sustained different selective pressures. The dog has adapted to life in human settlements, whereas the wolf has continued to survive relatively independently from man.

Domestication, then, is an historical process by which a species evolves in close association with man and thereby undergoes genetic changes in a direction desired by man. Selection takes place for the species just as it did in the wild, but instead of the "fittest" animals surviving, we might say that the "most desirable according to man" survive. That is, man actively intervenes in the selection process, deciding—to the extent that his technology allows him—which animals will be most highly prized, best cared for, and encouraged to reproduce.

Thus, because of the varied uses to which man has put his animals, traits which would be detrimental to survival in the wild sometimes actually enhance the survival chances of a domestic animal. White fur, for example, is a liability to most animals because it renders them conspicuous to predators or prey, but it may be highly valued by man. Because of this esthetic factor, domestic animals, especially those now bred for show, are often very different in appearance from their wild relatives.

Animals with the following characteristics have evidently been easiest to domesticate:

(1) They generally are adaptable to changed conditions. For example, unlike many zoo animals, they breed readily in captivity.

(2) They are generally social and hence interact rather easily with man. Even the solitary cat has a strong mother-offspring bond.

(3) They are usually hierarchical, rather than territorial, in their social organization. Hierarchical species readily travel with man and also are easy to lead, since they regard man as their superior and defer to his wishes. They also don't challenge his approach the way a territorial animal might. The territorial watchdog, bred for this tendency, might be regarded as the exception that proves the rule. However, most domestic animals are not aggressive, neither as individuals nor as species. They are accustomed to being dominated.

(4) They generally are promiscuous breeders, since if they were monogamous it would be difficult to breed them according to man's wishes.

(5) They usually eat a wide variety of foods. Many domestic species—dogs, cats, chickens, pigeons, and goats—are scavengers.

Although a species such as the dog has undergone this process of domestication, of digression from the wolf line, for about 10,000 years now, transition from the wild to the tame state, and vice versa, is surprisingly easy. Wolf cubs can easily be tamed, and feral dogs readily form a pack and survive in the wild.

A "tame" animal is one that, regardless of its historical association with or alienation from man, tolerates man's presence. Thus a circus or zoo lion may be tame or not, depending upon whether or not it has become accustomed to man during its lifetime. Animals on the Galapagos Islands, historically uninhabited by man, have not evolved a fear of man and hence do not have to undergo a taming process in order to tolerate him.

The essential criterion of tameness, then, is how closely the animal will allow man to approach it. In the wild, animals fear man and will flee when he gets within a reliably measurable "flight distance" from them. This fear can be gradually overcome in many animals, however, particularly young and, of course, domestic ones; that is, the flight distance can be progressively reduced to zero. This does not necessarily mean, however, that the animal will allow man to touch it. Only "contact" species will do so; "distance" species insist upon a degree of "individual distance" or personal space and won't let conspecifics brush against them either. In order to survive in captivity, an animal must at least become acclimated enough to let man approach it with food; that is, it must accept man's offerings of sustenance.

Domestic animals are usually tamed or socialized to man as a matter of course. However, if a domestic animal is kept rather isolated from man until maturity, it may have to be tamed or acclimated to man deliberately; this process is not always completely successful.

Captive animals should definitely be tamed, if possible, so that they are more manageable and so that their illnesses can be diagnosed and treated more effectively.

Animals, domestic or wild, are relatively easy to tame in infancy because man acts as a substitute parent toward them, as an object of imprinting. The first domesticated wolf cubs were probably tamed in this way. One side effect of this imprinting to man is that as an adult, the animal may regard humans as potential sex partners. However, the animal will usually prefer members of its own species, especially if it has been exposed to them during infancy.

Thus tameness has nothing to do with ferocity, except that an untamed animal that cannot maintain its flight distance from man, being cornered or otherwise feeling threatened, may attack. (The smallest, most innocuous animal will defend itself or its young as a last resort, but we would hardly call a cornered rabbit "ferocious.") Escaped untamed animals, then, are primarily concerned with avoiding man, not attacking him. This is all the more true because such escapees usually have been recently fed and would have to be very hungry indeed to overcome their hereditary fear of man and stalk him. Therefore, even the most powerful carnivores, if not threatened or abused, can be maneuvered back into captivity by personnel trained in the art of animal psychology.

Very often, in fact, escaped animals are anxious to return to their familiar surroundings and do not seem to regard themselves as prisoners. Many nonmigratory birds in zoos do not have to have their wings pinioned to prevent their flying away. And sometimes, tragically, an animal will return to its quarters even when they are aflame.

The animal's social bonds usually attract it to its habitat. At Munich's Hellabrun zoo, I was shocked to see a large male baboon scale the stone wall surrounding its rocky grounds. But rather than interact with the visitors, it ran round atop the wall and observed its troop, on one occasion quickly descending to bite a female to discipline her.

Tame animals may also be trained. Training consists of providing the animal with something to do. Training has been compared to human athletics or exercise; it keeps the organism fit. The extent to which animals need to be kept occupied is, however, debatable. Although a circus bear will occasionally be observed to ride a few laps on its bicycle spontaneously, adult animals have no well-established psychological need for activity. A wild lion, for example, is content to remain almost motionless for days if well fed. Young animals do, however, show a decided interest in play; this activity probably is instrumental in their learning how to run, hunt, or whatever. A cleverly trained, well-conditioned animal is, however, indisputably more attractive than a fat, inert one. And it is less likely to be hypersexual, antisocial, or to engage in stereotyped movement.

Just as captive animals require little exercise to survive, they need little space. Zoo animals usually far outlive their wild brethren, due in part to the relative ease of cleaning and disinfecting a small, smooth cage floor. However, birds and other animals sometimes require room enough to perform courtship displays and to mate, if they are to reproduce. (An animal's ability to reproduce is regarded as the best proof that it has been properly treated.)

Animals are usually tamed, then, by a human being acting as a parent to the young animal. And they are trained by a human being acting as a superior, rewarding and punishing their behavior appropriately. But even though an animal's owner may intimidate it, other people may not. Thus, for example, a dog's master must take advantage of his status with his pet to train it not to bite anyone. Most attacks by dogs and other animals are due to the animal's feeling that its social status or territory is being challenged by a rival.

Animals are, of course, capable of amazing feats of intelligence. But their behavior with regard to their masters can border on the incredible also, and can only be comprehended by bearing in mind the special nature of the relationship. Animals have often been known to defend their masters from other animals, and even to help retrieve errant animals. But they have also been observed to cower behind their masters when threatened by another animal. Circus animals occasionally even discipline other animals that fail to perform their tricks properly.

Another surprising aspect of animal psychology concerns priority of access to a space. The first animal to occupy a cage frequently defends the territory against later arrivals, so that it is advisable to introduce all of the residents of a cage at the same time. This same principle explains why an animal trainer enters the cage first and ostentatiously occupies the center in a confident, unhesitating manner: he is establishing his dominance. (The reason why cages and circus rings are usually circular is so that the animals are less prone to try to establish a nook of the space as their own domain.) Because they are easy to dominate, subordinate animals are usually the easiest to train. They may even come to depend upon their trainer to keep more dominant animals from bullying them. And since illness usually lowers an animal's rank, sick animals are often strongly attached to man. This attraction can be turned to advantage in ministering to the animal.

Association with man has many important effects on an animal, and where reproductive behavior is affected, future generations and hence genetic makeup are altered inevitably. In the case of domestic animals, man attempts to control these genetic changes, to improve his stock in accordance with his needs. But in the case of zoo and laboratory animals, man's goal is to retain wild type genes so that he can observe and study the animals as they have evolved in nature.

For practical reasons, man tries to get these wild animals to reproduce in captivity, by simulating their natural environment in essential respects. Nevertheless, man's interference is unavoidable and necessarily affects the characteristics of surviving offspring. For example, zoo animals often breed at the wrong time of year so that the young are born during the winter; such offspring would not survive in the wild but they usually do in captivity. Similarly, Norway rats have been domesticated for use in laboratory experiments, but these laboratory animals are considerably gentler than the original stock, because experimenters obviously prefer to handle more docile animals.

It seems unavoidable, then, for man to distort the behavior of any captive animal. If the animal cannot be made to reproduce, obviously it is not behaving naturally. And if the animal can be made to reproduce in captivity, man's interference inexorably affects the selective process, simply because even the most modern, naturalistic zoos and animal parks are only simulations of natural milieux. For example, zoo animals often reach sexual maturity precociously, come into heat irregularly due to unnatural lighting or unwonted climate, have unusually large litters, and engage in sex either unusually often or unusually seldom. These and other factors affect the genetic makeup of succeeding generations.

In order to appreciate animals for what, or who, they are, man must try to minimize his interference and maximize the naturalness of the animal's surroundings. Animals should be taught, to the extent possible, to tolerate man's approach. But man, and particularly children, should be taught that close contact with an animal is not necessarily the best way to learn about or to treat it. Animals can never be made to think as people do, and the better we understand these differences, the more satisfaction we can derive from our interactions with them.

The field of ethology, the study of animals in nature, is making fascinating discoveries that carry intriguing implications for human behavior. Animals have always captivated man, but now, through an application of modern biological principles, we are beginning to understand not just what things animals do but why they do them, what survival value their behavior patterns have. Thus we can do more than just admire an animal's beauty, grace, or intelligence; we can understand why it looks or behaves as it does. If it has wide-set eyes with horizontal pupils, we can infer that it is a prey species equipped to view the entire horizon for predators. If its teeth are large and flat like millstones, we know that it is a herbivore adapted for grinding up tough plant food. If the male and female of the species are very similar in appearance, their behavior is probably similar and so they may both care for the young and hence be monogamous.

Included in the list of books at the end of this chapter are recommended introductions to animal, not just pet, behavior. Domestic animals can best be understood by first applying the general principles of behavior to their actions, and by considering how their ancestral species must have lived in the wild. Modifications of behavior through domestication are usually minor.

The same kind of inferences can, of course, be made with regard to human behavior. The great part of hominid evolution took place when man hunted meat and gathered plants and lived in groups of perhaps a hundred individuals. Much of human anatomy and behavior only makes sense when considered in that ecological context. Thus the study of animal behavior patterns in terms of function and survival value provides a key to understanding our own bodies and feelings. Our great interest in animals is itself doubtless inherent, in that man needed to know about predators and sources of meat in order to survive. At the same time that we indulge this interest, we also inevitably learn about the living world and our place within it.

DOGS

Domestic dogs, it is believed, are descended from wolf-like canids, possibly with an admixture of jackal blood in some strains. Selective breeding has resulted in the emphasis of certain traits found in the modern wolf, and the de-emphasis of others. Dogs are generally smaller, more docile, and less sociable toward each other than are wolves. Perhaps because man is inherently attracted by infantile features, dogs apparently have been bred for puppy-like traits such as floppy ears, short legs, short muzzles, and small teeth. These immature characteristics also occur in wolf cubs but are lost in the adult wolf. But the point is often made that man, in domesticating the dog, did not introduce any fundamentally new traits, but rather simply played up traits which were already present in wolves. The fundamental similarity of canids is borne out by the fact that dogs, wolves, foxes, coyotes, and jackals can usually interbreed and can be tamed readily, at least when young.

Behavioral as well as anatomical traits reflect the dog's ancestry. Retrieving bones is a throwback to the canid habit of bringing back to the den meat from the hunt for injured, young, or lactating members of the pack. This propensity has, of course, been exploited in dogs bred as retrievers. Like other canids, dogs scent-mark their territories. This less desirable habit is probably inseparable from the dog's territorial nature, which man utilizes in guard dogs. And canids are willing to eat almost anything, a characteristic that probably led to the domestication of the dog originally; wolves presumably scavenged around human settlements and were gradually drafted for other functions. Wolves have been known to dig up human corpses in recent times.

Canids are highly social animals, and their capacity for hunting cooperatively is one of the chief factors favoring their domestication. Cooperation means taking advantage of both force of numbers and specialization of roles. A pack of canids can hunt even large animals successfully not just because they can gang up on the prey but also because they can specialize in particular aspects of the hunt. Some wolves in the pack seem especially proficient at running down the prey, while others customarily attack the neck and still others the hindquarters. These idiosyncrasies, which even serve to distinguish littermates, have provided man with the leverage necessary to selectively breed dogs for coursing, tracking, herding, and attacking game, as well as for other purposes.

The canid pack, then, is diversified. This permits not only role specialization but also leadership, in that the pack members must subordinate their efforts to a single cooperative aim. This capacity for obedience is assumed to account for the dog's trainability. Naturally, this means that the dog must accept its master as dominant over it.

The dog is man's oldest friend, having been domesticated before the caribou and all other animals. The hundreds of breeds, reflecting the great variety of the wolf gene pool, have been used for dozens of purposes, including turning water wheels, pulling or carrying burdens, carrying messages, scouting, trailing suspected criminals, and fighting in gladiatorial contests. Dogs have been used for food and their hides for clothing, and they have been used in sacrificial ceremonies. Dogs were raised as pets and given names by the ancient Egyptians. Later, the toy breeds were developed as pets. Their small size and short muzzles appeal to our inherent attraction to "cute," infantile features. Dogs have also been used for massed attacks in warfare and are still trained for police work. In recent times, dogs have been put to new uses as laboratory animals and as guide dogs for the blind.

Their principal uses, however, have been in hunting, herding, and guarding.

Originally, dogs did most of the killing of game as well as the tracking and coursing. The Afghan breed, for example, was developed in the Sinai desert and later in mountainous regions. These dogs were trained to hunt in pairs, one dog attacking the throat and the other the hindquarters, in the manner of wolves. The adult's warm coat protects it against the cold of Asia, but the puppy's short hair betrays the Afghan's derivation from the greyhound group and desert climes. Afghans and salukis can hurdle and dodge rocks while maintaining speed.

Dogs, of course, can be trained to be excellent trackers. Only the scent of an identical twin target—and sometimes not even that—can throw off a well-trained tracking dog. When tracking humans in police work, the dog relies upon scents released by disturbances in the ground or vegetation (these, however, being nonspecific to the target), as well as those emanating from the target's body and clothing.

The dog's herding instincts derive from the wolf's ability to drive animals over cliffs, and this technique was formerly used by domesticated dogs when man was hunting game on a large scale. Sheep dogs must, however, treat their charges gently, and so they merely "show-eye" or stare them back in place. Because "shepherd" dogs were responsible for guarding as well as herding animals, they were bred for loyalty to a single master. This tendency is still apparent in collies, German shepherds, and English sheep dogs.

Dog breeds are often classified by function rather than descent, for the reason that dogs of diverse origin have been bred for similar purposes, and also because dog breeds are really not very distinct genetically. However, the following classification probably has some validity.

The dingo line, a primitive type of dog, probably originated in

India. These semidomesticated dogs, found today in Australia, Africa, and the Far East, are often attached to human settlements as scavengers. They may be regarded, both behaviorally and anatomically, as exemplifying an intermediate position in the evolution of the fully domesticated dog. They are cringing and fearful. They have large, primitive teeth. They have no dew claw on the hind limb (those of modern dogs, generally removed surgically at birth, represent a vestigial fifth digit). They do not bark in the wild, although they can learn to do so. And they go into estrus only once a year, in autumn, as wild canids do.

The greyhound line was probably developed in southern desert regions. These dogs have been used for running down animals. Modern greyhounds can reach a speed of 37 miles per hour (60 kilometers per hour). They are found in Scotland and Ireland (no one knows how they got there), and from North Africa to Russia and Afghanistan.

The mastiffs seem to have developed in the mountainous regions stretching from the Himalayas to the Pyrenees. They are characterized by exceptional powers of scent, silky coats, large floppy ears, and short muzzles. They were bred principally as shepherd dogs, their courage and fierceness being useful in guarding flocks. Modern breeds, however, are quite companionable and affectionate. But the terriers remain remarkably aggressive. These breeds were developed for burrowing into the ground (French *terre*) in pursuit of game and vermin. Digging, of course, comes naturally to the lair-dwelling canids. The lineage of terriers is uncertain.

The northern group, including dogs known as "spitz," are closely related to the large grey wolves of Europe. Eskimos, in fact, continue to breed back their huskies to wild wolves. These dogs were used for pulling sledges and for herding and guarding animals, including caribou. Wolves can separate a single animal out from a herd, an ability exploited in these breeds, which include elkhounds, collies, and German shepherds.

Dog behavior unfolds along the following lines. The newborn puppy is blind and deaf but can locate the nipple and suckle by means of olfactory and tactile reflexes. If a puppy must be bottle-fed, it should be supported on a warm, soft surface and the nipple must not be forcefully inserted. The idea is to conform to the puppy's innate behavior patterns.

Puppies have been found to utter distinctive cries for signaling the mother that they are (1) being lain upon or in danger of falling; (2) cold; (3) hot; and (4) retaining urine or feces. For the first 2½ weeks of life, the mother's licking is usually required to stimulate urination and defecation. She then swallows the puppy's feces; this keeps the nest clean and also makes it more difficult for a potential predator to detect. I once knew a female dog that showed an extreme form of this trait, patrolling the entire neighborhood like an inspired sanitation crew.

After 2½ weeks, the puppy leaves the whelping box to excrete. Later on, at about 8 weeks, puppies tend to concentrate their efforts on a particular area of the kennel. This obviously is adaptive for a lair-dwelling species and apparently is related to the adult male habit of scent-marking spots where animals have excreted previously. This tendency can be utilized in housebreaking a puppy, by leading it to the desired spot repeatedly. Naturally it is very helpful to have the dog excrete initially on newspaper or in some other desirable location. The dog's eliminative behavior pattern seems to require some preliminary moving around, so if the puppy is confined to its sleeping box overnight, it usually will not soil it. Until it is 12 weeks old, however, a puppy is likely to urinate or defecate every hour or two, while awake.

The social order of the litter is established from about the 4th week until the time of weaning, at 8 to 10 weeks. In order to take advantage of this period of socialization, the owner is advised to take the puppy home by about 6 to 8 weeks.

Beginning at about 4 weeks, some females may regurgitate solid food for their puppies, as wolf parents do.

During the "critical period" for socialization, the dominance order of the litter is determined. The puppies fight to decide which of them will get priority of access to food and other resources. This order remains rather stable into adulthood. Highly aggressive breeds such as basenjis and wirehaired fox terriers have closed, rigid hierarchies, and males usually dominate females. Terrier puppies often gang up on each other and have to be broken up into small groups. Cocker spaniels, however, are less competitive. They are more open to newcomers and gender is less important in determining rank.

The relative status of two dogs can often be inferred from their postures. Dominant dogs—and mammals in general—carry themselves proudly or conspicuously, with heads and tails high. Subordinate animals are downcast and avoid the gaze of the superordinate. The submissive posture of canids consists of lying on one's back, perhaps derived from the puppies' position for being licked and similarly inhibiting attack. Licking a person's face is probably a submissive gesture derived from the infantile (and hence nonthreatening) behavior pattern of lapping up food regurgitated by adult dogs. Tail-wagging is a friendly, submissive gesture, in most circumstances, and has apparently been selected for by man. The dog's open-mouthed grin, with flattened ears, extruded tongue, and wagging tail, is an expression given to humans but not to other dogs. It may have evolved because man finds it so appealing.

Dogs are territorial as well as hierarchical animals, as their scent-marking implies. A scientist once demonstrated this canid propensity to demarcate an individual territory by devoting an evening to drinking tea and urinating over a portion of a wolf's territory. The wolf then generously withdrew his boundary outside of the territory established by the man. Dogs, of course, regard their master's house and property as their den and territory, and defend them against intruders. Dogs that are kept tied up may be especially aggressive because this attachment to a particular location has been intensified.

The period from 4 to 11 weeks is the time when the dog is sensitive to training as well as socialization. Dogs kept isolated from human contact during this time are difficult to tame later on. The essential step in socializing a puppy is to establish dominance over it. One very effective means of doing so is to lift the puppy and shake it punitively by the scruff of the neck. The neck in many mammals, being the object of most predatory attacks, is a well-protected yet highly sensitive area. Many species, notably the opossum, when grabbed by the neck will go into a "death feint," pretending to be unpalatable to the predator. This response has apparently been "emancipated" or recruited in the course of evolution for use in other behavioral contexts. For example, female mammals often carry their young by the neck, contact there rendering them passive. And in many species the male grasps the female in the neck region during mating; presumably this too takes advantage of the animal's passive reaction to such stimulation. Another such region, incidentally, is the loin area. Nursing females relax and hold still when touched in this area, for obvious reasons; and the male often grasps the female around the waist during mating. For additional evidence of this response, consider the fact that the nape of the neck and the waist of women are regarded as erogenous zones.

To return to the original point, the owner should establish dominance over the puppy. And if he wants the dog to be friendly toward people in general, he should have many different individuals handle it during the socialization period.

Puppies can be trained using a variety of reinforcers: hitting, praise (remarkably effective on dogs), shaking by the neck, petting, and solitary confinement (dogs are very vulnerable to loneliness). Experiments have shown that dogs can actually learn to respond to particular words and not just to their master's tone of voice. Dogs can, of course, be trained to do extraordinary things, including climbing ladders.

Dogs continue to grow into the second year. They reach sexual maturity considerably earlier than wolves—usually in the first year for females and sometimes a while later in males, depending upon the breed. As with other mammals, mating is facilitated if the male is dominant over the female. It also helps if the male is on familiar territory. Spayed females are generally nonreceptive. Intact females come into estrus twice a year, at no particular season. At this time they bleed slightly from the vagina; this is unrelated to the phenomenon of menstruation. The urine of estrous females attracts males, but the female does not become receptive until the latter part of the estrous period, when bleeding has ended. The functional significance of the copulatory tie is unknown, except that ejaculation continues while the dogs remain coupled.

Dogs reach senescence at from 7 to 12 years, depending upon the breed.

CATS

The domestic cat is probably descended from the bush cat *Felis lysica* of Africa, with an admixture from the European cat *F. sylvestris*. Cats have been used for killing rodents, for help in retrieving game, and as pets. As is well known, they were revered and mummified by the ancient Egyptians.

When kittens are very young, they cry when separated from their mother, who then usually retrieves them. At 5 weeks they begin to follow her when she goes to feed or, in the wild, hunt. In this way they can learn by observation. The mother effectively teaches her kittens by performing fragments of predatory behavior—catching the prey but not killing it, for example—so as to provide opportunities for practicing the omitted steps. However, the mother's behavior is quite stereotyped and inappropriate at times; she apparently doesn't know what she is doing and hence cannot be regarded as much of a teacher. But sometimes she mews when the kitten desists from practicing its predation, and this seems to encourage it to resume its lesson.

Kittens can be weaned at about 6 weeks if they are eating milk and meat from dishes at that time.

As is commonly said, kittens are independent animals. They do not socialize much among themselves. After puberty they play much less than before, especially the females. The more active of two cats is usually the dominant one, but dominance is not a very significant phenomenon in this species. Some males do, however, show marked territoriality.

Yowling is a male courtship display. Males reach sexual maturity at 8 to 15 months of age.

Females reach puberty at 6 to 8 months. They have two breeding seasons in temperate climates, in early spring and early fall. In warmer climates or when exposed artificially to longer daily periods of light, they have three or four seasons annually. Each breeding season has several estrous periods of anywhere from 4 to 10 days, the period being longer if the cat remains unmated. A cat in heat will exhibit hindleg treading and lordosis (arching of the back) if its neck skin is grasped, its back is rubbed, and its anogenital region is patted at the same time.

Unlike canids, cats hunt mainly by sound and sight, and at night. Their narrow pupillary slits widen in darkness to admit the maximum of light. And, like most nocturnal animals, they have a tapetum behind the retina to reflect light back to the photosensitive cells and thus magnify its intensity. This mirror-like structure is what makes a cat's eyes seem to glow in the dark and may explain why the animal has long been regarded as a source of special powers. Cats also hear high frequencies very well, possibly so that they can detect the cries of rodents. This may account for the fact that they seem to respond more to a woman's voice than to a man's.

Cats hunt by ambush or by stalking. If a cat detects a likely target, it runs toward it noiselessly, belly close to the ground: the "stalking run." The cat then pauses, stalks slowly, and finally pounces on its victim with unsheathed claws, usually biting the neck simultaneously. The cat then leaves the area, returning shortly to carry off its prey to a secluded place for consumption.

Experiments have been performed to determine the extent to which killing of rodents is untutored in cats. Kittens raised with females that were given occasional opportunities to kill rodents killed them, as adult cats, much more readily than did kittens that had never seen an animal killed. Kittens raised with rodents as cagemates later never killed the type of animal—rat or mouse —with which they had been raised. When presented with a rodent in the test situation, they often treated it as a playmate. Like all other forms of complex behavior, predation in cats is shaped by experience as well as by a gentically-determined behavioral substrate.

Predatory behavior does not seem to be enhanced by raising a kitten on meat as opposed to a vegetarian diet, but it does affect whether or not the cat will eat the prey that it kills. If a farm cat is kept to control rodents, it is advisable, in fact, to feed it regularly, in order to keep it attached to the farm.

Indeed, many cats do go feral, living as scavengers in cities or retreating to rural areas. Their secretive habits probably result in our underestimating their numbers. They are not as divorced from their wild ancestors as are dogs, and they survive very well on their own.

When domestic cats breed in the wild state, their appearance, generally speaking, reverts to the wild tabby coloring. All other fur patterns and colors represent mutant forms favored only by selective breeding.

HORSES

The horse evolved from a four-toed shrub-eater into a hoofed prairie-dweller with longer legs and stronger jaws and teeth. It evolved in North America and then migrated to Asia, Europe, and Africa. It then became extinct in the New World until reintroduced by the Spanish. The only surviving wild horse is the now-rare Przewalski's horse discovered in 1881 in Mongolia. Another subspecies, the tarpan, was depicted in Paleolithic cave paintings but disappeared as a distinct entity in 1851.

The horse was first used for drawing carts and war chariots, and only later for riding. Originally domesticated by the tribes of the steppes of Southern Russia and central Asia, the horse was probably responsible for the development of nomadic life and for the successful invasion by barbaric Indo-European nomads of the more civilized regions to the south.

Horses exhibit sundry bits of interesting behavior. They can be trained to track lost cows in the manner of a hunting dog. They defecate in a particular part of the field where they do not graze. In winter they roll in the mud to apply a protective layer against the weather. In spring they shed their winter coats.

Horses often sleep, standing up, during the hottest part of the day. But one horse usually remains alert as a look-out. Darker horses are less vigilant, as a rule, than lighter ones. This may be due to their being less conspicuous; *viz.* the genes for color and vigilance may have been selected as a unit. Grey horses, being especially cautious, often warn the herd of an approaching stranger. This does not mean, however, that such a horse necessarily leads the herd in other situations.

A stallion usually leads the herd, and males generally dominate females. Age and size are also factors enhancing superiority. Dominance contests are fought with the teeth and the fore hooves. Among horses running wild, one group often dominates a smaller neighboring group.

When two horses meet for the first time, they follow a regular sequence of introduction: (1) they circle around each other; (2) they touch nostrils; (3) they investigate each other's tails and bodies with their noses; and (4) if mutual tolerance is decided upon, they nibble each other along the crest of the neck. If the animals are close in social rank, a dominance struggle may ensue.

"Wither-nibbling" usually indicates recognition. It is often seen when two horses meet after a separation. "Friends" are usually close in social rank, as is the case in other species.

If a single horse is attacked by a predator, it will usually defend itself with its hind hooves. But a herd of feral horses, when alarmed, will sometimes form a line shoulder-to-shoulder.

Wild horses have a breeding season, with several estrous periods, but domestic horses are receptive all year round. However, in some domestic individuals and breeds, ovulation accompanies estrus only during the breeding season and so there is a limited foaling season, about 11 months later, in the spring, when births are most likely to take place. Each estrous period lasts about 5 to 9 days.

The lens of the equine eye is nonelastic. The animal focuses by raising or lowering its head to bring the image onto the appropriate part of the sloping retina. The eyeball is shaped in such a way that when the horse is grazing, both near objects on the ground and distant ones on the horizon are in focus simultaneously.

Untamed horses will allow themselves to be touched on the neck, withers, and back but not on other parts. The legs and feet are the last members that a horse will let be touched. No matter how tame, a zebra usually will not allow its feet to be touched; consequently, the hooves can only be medicated after anesthetizing the animal.

A horse's mood can be discerned by paying attention to auditory and visual cues.

A snort often means danger. Neighing indicates excitement; it occurs in distress, as when the horse gets separated from its companions, and in male courtship. The whinny indicates close communication or courtship.

As with most mammals, if a horse sets its ears back, it is ready to defend itself. A lashing tail presages a kick. A raised head and waving upper lip sometimes imply nausea.

Horses are not noted for their powers of reasoning. They will, for example, have great difficulty finding their way by an indirect route through a couple of gates when they have become separated from their companions.

On the other hand, horses are extremely sensitive to subtle sensory cues. The "Clever Hans" case illustrates this. Hans was a performing horse that appeared to answer arithmetic problems by tapping out the correct solution with his hoof. It was eventually discovered, however, that Hans was actually only responding to his trainer's inadvertent anticipatory movements when Hans got to the correct number of taps. Hans's performances were hardly less clever for being fraudulent—especially when compared to the intelligence of the audiences whom he deceived.

Training horses is generally regarded as a fine art, but several principles can be articulated.

A young horse should never be overworked; it should be allowed to absorb what it has just been taught.

The trainer should make an effort to understand the horse's characteristic facial expressions.

Signals should be given consistently, since horses are sensitive to tone of voice, slight movements, and subtle pressure. This may be why horses are anxious under a tense rider.

Horses should not be taught by trial and error, but rather by shaping their responses in the desired direction. For example, if the horse is being taught to respond to its name, the name should be uttered and the horse pulled forward and given food as a reward. Repetition of such performances establishes the desired habit.

Racehorse training consists mainly of exercise: building up the animal's speed and stamina. Horses differ greatly in their dependence on the jockey for guidance during a race. Much of a horse's success rests on the confidence it has acquired in previous contests. A horse often remembers its earlier experience on a given track, as shown by the fact that it may tense up at the spot of a previous fall, or it may speed up where it did the last time around.

Horses can exhibit forms of undesirable behavior, or "vices," such as the following:

The horse rears in order to evade forward action; for example, a horse may rear in an attempt to throw off the rider. This is a sign of anxiety, so it is best to calm the horse rather than try to punish it. Most vices are, in fact, due to anxiety, not to perverseness, and usually develop as a result of confinement or loneliness.

Bolting means that the horse does not stop when ordered to do so. The first instance is usually due to fear, but bolting may become habitual. A more severe bit can be employed, but it is often best to reschool the horse to vocal signals.

A horse that jibs is one that refuses to go forward. Its confidence may be augmented by rewards and by firmness on the part of the rider. When the horse does move on (another horse's example often helps), it should then be returned to the original spot and the procedure should be repeated.

A horse may bite when girthed up or groomed under the abdomen. A softer brush may help, but a muzzle may be called for.

A horse usually kicks its stable out of boredom. If the stable is padded and the animal can no longer make a racket, the fun seems to go out of the activity, and the habit usually disappears.

SUGGESTED READING

W. Etkin, *Social Behavior from Fish to Man.* University of Chicago Press (ppr.), 1967.

E. S. E. Hafez (ed.), *The Behavior of Domestic Animals.* Baltimore: Williams & Wilkins Co., 1976 (3rd ed.).

H. Hediger, *The Psychology and Behavior of Animals in Zoos and Circuses.* New York: Dover Publications (ppr.), 1968.

J. Sparks, *Bird Behaviour.* London: Hamlyn Publishing Group (ppr.), 1969.

D. G. Freedman, *Human Infancy: An Evolutionary Perspective.* Hillsdale, N.J.: Lawrence Erlbaum Associates, 1974.